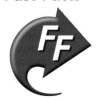

Fast Facts

KU-505-602

Fast Facts:
Asthma

Second edition

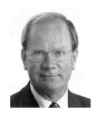

Stephen T Holgate MD DSc FRCP FMedSci
MRC Clinical Professor of Immunopharmacology
School of Medicine
Southampton General Hospital
Southampton, UK

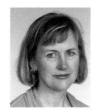

Jo Douglass MB BS MD FRACP
Head, Allergy, Asthma and Clinical Immunology Service
Alfred Hospital and Monash University
Melbourne, Victoria, Australia

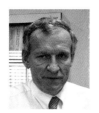

This book is dedicated to the memory of
Romain A Pauwels
Professor at the Department of Respiratory Diseases
University Hospital, Ghent, Belgium, who co-wrote the first
edition and contributed to early drafts of this edition

Declaration of Independence
This book is as balanced and as practical as
we can make it. Ideas for improvement are
always welcome: feedback@fastfacts.com

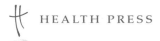

HEALTH PRESS

Fast Facts: Asthma
First published 1999
Second edition October 2006

Text © 2006 Stephen T Holgate, Jo Douglass
© 2006 in this edition Health Press Limited

Health Press Limited, Elizabeth House, Queen Street, Abingdon,
Oxford OX14 3LN, UK
Tel: +44 (0)1235 523233
Fax: +44 (0)1235 523238

Book orders can be placed by telephone or via the website.
For regional distributors or to order via the website, please go to:
www.fastfacts.com
For telephone orders, please call 01752 202301 (UK), +44 1752 202301 (Europe),
1 800 247 6553 (USA, toll free) or +1 419 281 1802 (Americas).

Fast Facts is a trademark of Health Press Limited.

All rights reserved. No part of this publication may be reproduced, stored
in a retrieval system, or transmitted in any form or by any means, electronic,
mechanical, photocopying, recording or otherwise, without the express
permission of the publisher.

The rights of Stephen T Holgate and Jo Douglass to be identified as the authors of
this work have been asserted in accordance with the Copyright,
Designs & Patents Act 1988 Sections 77 and 78.

The publisher and the authors have made every effort to ensure the accuracy of this
book, but cannot accept responsibility for any errors or omissions.

For all drugs, please consult the product labeling approved in your country for
prescribing information.

Registered names, trademarks, etc. used in this book, even when not marked as such,
are not to be considered unprotected by law.

A CIP record for this title is available from the British Library.

ISBN 1-903734-54-1 (978-1-903734-54-4)

Holgate ST (Stephen)
Fast Facts: Asthma/
Stephen T Holgate, Jo Douglass

Medical illustrations by Dee McLean and Jane Fallows,
Medee Art, London, UK.
Typesetting and page layout by Zed, Oxford, UK.
Printed by LinneyPrint Ltd, Mansfield, UK.

Text printed with vegetable inks on fully biodegradable and
recyclable paper manufactured from sustainable forests.

444   001
Low emissions
during production

Low
chlorine

Sustainable
forests

Glossary

AMP: adenosine 5'-monophosphate

Atopy: a condition characterized by excessive production of IgE in response to allergens

Basophil: a type of white blood cell, distinguishable on staining

B lymphocyte: a type of white blood cell that produces antibodies

COPD: chronic obstructive pulmonary disease

CysLTs: cysteinyl leukotrienes, a powerful class of bronchoconstricting mediators

Cytokine: a peptide secreted by cells involved in inflammation and the immune response. Cytokines can control the activity and growth of the cell that secreted them, or nearby cells

Daily variability: variability in daily peak expiratory flow (PEF), calculated as a percentage of the mean daily PEF value

DPI: dry-powder inhaler

Eosinophil: a type of white blood cell involved in allergic responses, distinguishable on staining

FEV$_1$: forced expiratory volume in 1 second, a measure of lung function

FVC: forced vital capacity, a measure of lung function

GINA: Global Initiative for Asthma, an international scientific initiative created to provide and encourage the use of scientific reports on asthma and asthma research

IgE: immunoglobulin class E, a class of antibody secreted by B lymphocytes on exposure to allergen. Binding of IgE to certain cells involved in the immune response results in the release of inflammatory mediators

IL: interleukin, a cytokine that controls a specific aspect of hemopoiesis or the immune response

IL-2: interleukin-2, a cytokine that stimulates T lymphocytes during the immune response

IL-2R: interleukin-2 receptor, expressed on activated T lymphocytes

Interferon-γ: a cytokine that has the capacity to inhibit the development of the allergic pathways, under normal conditions

LABA: long-acting β$_2$-agonist

Leukocyte: white blood cell

Mast cell: a large cell containing chemical mediators that are released in inflammatory and allergic responses

MDI: metered-dose inhaler

PaO$_2$: partial pressure of oxygen in arterial blood

PaCO$_2$: partial pressure of carbon dioxide in arterial blood

PEF: peak expiratory flow, a measure of lung function

pMDI: pressurized metered-dose inhaler

SaO$_2$: oxygen saturation in arterial blood

T lymphocyte: a type of white blood cell that is mainly responsible for cell-mediated immunity

T_H lymphocyte: T-helper lymphocyte. Type of T lymphocyte that is activated on exposure to allergen and releases cytokines

Trigger: a stimulus that increases asthma symptoms and/or airflow limitation

Introduction

Studies throughout the world have clearly demonstrated that asthma and allied allergic disorders are increasing in incidence and possibly in severity. This is reflected not only by epidemiological studies, but also by hospital admissions and the use of medication. While it has long been recognized that asthma is a disorder of widespread airway obstruction, reversible either spontaneously or with treatment, research over the past decade has reaffirmed that underlying airway inflammation is the predominant cause of the airway dysfunction. As asthma is a chronic inflammatory disease, structural changes also occur in the airways, leading to increased responsiveness to a variety of stimuli and, over time, possibly the gradual deterioration of pulmonary function. Asthma most commonly begins in early childhood, and the condition may last a lifetime. Like all chronic inflammatory diseases, its severity may vary from mild and intermittent to severe and persistent. Thus, its impact on the quality of life of an individual can vary through life. However, if asthma is correctly diagnosed and properly treated, most patients can lead a normal life, although many will need to take medications regularly to do so.

Attacks of asthma have, in the past, led physicians to treat the disease as a series of acute episodes rather than as a chronic relapsing and remitting disorder. For this reason national and international guidelines for asthma management have been developed that focus on diagnosis, assessment of severity and objective measures, prevention, adequate drug treatment, patient education associated with self-management strategies, and appropriate follow-up. *Fast Facts: Asthma* draws its information from the Global Initiative for Asthma (GINA) guidelines, a document produced in collaboration with the World Health Organization and the US National Heart Lung and Blood Institute. In this book, we have attempted to distill the essential features of the latest GINA guidelines into a palatable and easily accessible form without losing information.

By the time guidelines for any disease are written and published they are, almost by definition, out of date on account of the continued research into the disease and its management. Asthma is no exception. However, mechanisms have now been developed to update guidelines more regularly, and they will be based more and more on newly published evidence and less on consensus. Where asthma guidelines have been introduced and disseminated and their findings have been taken up, the national indices for morbidity and mortality are showing declining trends.

It is our intention that this book provide the basis for good asthma management. However, guidelines are guidelines, and should not be taken as rules. The individual patient must be assessed in his or her own right, with individual circumstances taken into account. The principles raised in this book should nevertheless provide a framework to improve the lives of the many patients who suffer from this disease.

Romain Pauwels, the co-author of the previous edition of this book, died in 2005. He was a keen advocate of evidence-based medicine and made a large contribution in his lifetime to improved asthma care for patients. We dedicate this edition to him in recognition of the fact that he championed better provision of information about asthma to the public.

Asthma is a chronic inflammatory condition of the airways. It is characterized by recurrent episodes of airflow limitation, which, depending on the severity of the attack, produce symptoms such as breathlessness, wheezing, chest tightness and cough. Acute exacerbations can be rapid or gradual in onset, and may be severe and potentially life-threatening.

Autopsy studies of patients who have died from asthma show hyperinflated lungs, with both large and small airways blocked by plugs containing a mixture of mucus, serum proteins, inflammatory cells and cell debris. Microscopic examination reveals extensive inflammatory infiltration of the airways (Figure 1.1), with edema

Thickened mucosa   Plug of mucus, cells and debris   Thickened sub-basement membrane collagen

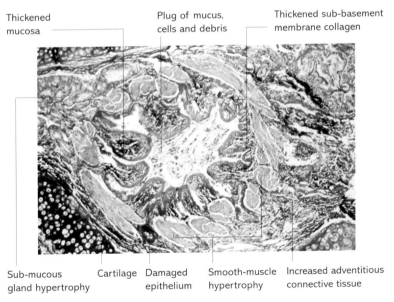

Sub-mucous gland hypertrophy   Cartilage   Damaged epithelium   Smooth-muscle hypertrophy   Increased adventitious connective tissue

Figure 1.1 Pathological features associated with death from asthma. Airways are blocked by plugs of mucus and inflammatory exudate. There is also vasodilatation and edema, vascular remodeling, smooth-muscle hypertrophy, and thickening of the basement membrane.

due to vasodilatation and blood vessel engorgement, and epithelial disruption. Biopsy studies have shown increased numbers of leukocytes, particularly eosinophils, mast cells and T lymphocytes, in the airways, and increases in the markers of lymphocyte activation. Structural changes resulting from chronic inflammation include bronchial smooth-muscle hypertrophy and hyperplasia, new vessel formation, interstitial collagen deposition resulting in basement membrane thickening, and airway wall remodeling.

Disease mechanisms

In most cases, asthma is an allergic disorder mediated, in part, by immunoglobulin E (IgE)-dependent mechanisms. Exposure to allergen results in allergen uptake and presentation by dendritic cells, activation of T-helper (T_H) lymphocytes, cytokine release from T_H cells, and secretion of specific IgE antibodies from B lymphocytes (Figure 1.2). IgE binds to mast cells and, possibly,

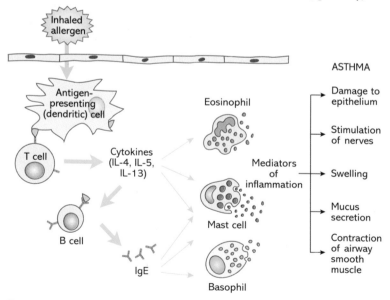

Figure 1.2 Role of immunoglobulin E (IgE) in airway inflammation and asthma symptoms. Exposure to allergen leads to activation of T lymphocytes, cytokine expression (interleukins [ILs]) and release of IgE from B lymphocytes. IgE binds to cells involved in inflammation, which then release inflammatory mediators.

other cells involved in inflammation (e.g. eosinophils), leading to the release of inflammatory mediators. In addition, exposure to antigens can provoke T-cell activation, cytokine and chemokine release, and production of inflammatory mediators by IgE-independent mechanisms.

Chronic inflammation is responsible for the two principal manifestations of disordered lung function in asthma: bronchial hyperresponsiveness and acute limitation of airflow (Table 1.1). Patients with asthma show an enhanced bronchoconstrictor response to a variety of stimuli such as histamine and methacholine (direct airway smooth-muscle stimuli), and exercise, adenosine monophosphate (AMP) and cold or dry air (indirect stimuli), causing airway narrowing secondary to the release of inflammatory mediators. This results in an increased variability in airway diameter and, therefore, in measures of lung function such as peak expiratory flow (PEF; Figure 1.3). Characteristically in asthma, PEF varies by more than 20% between morning and evening measurements.

In asthmatic airways, reductions in airflow can be due to acute bronchoconstriction, swelling of the airway wall, chronic mucous plugging or airway wall remodeling. Acute bronchoconstriction may occur as a result of allergen-induced release of inflammatory

TABLE 1.1

Manifestations of disordered lung function in asthma

- Airway hyperresponsiveness
- Airflow limitation
    - acute bronchoconstriction
    - swelling of the airway wall
    - chronic mucus plug formation
    - airway wall remodeling
- Stimulation of neurons
    - cough
    - chest tightness

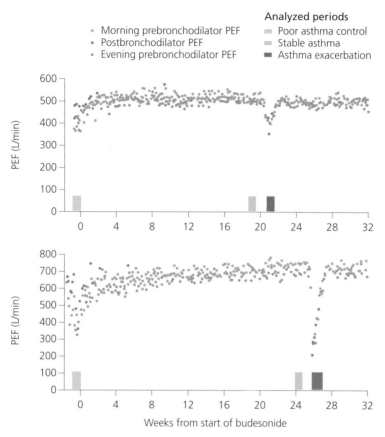

Figure 1.3 Peak expiratory flow (PEF), with and without budesonide treatment, showing within-day and between-day variations and exacerbations for 2 patients.

mediators such as histamine, prostaglandins and leukotrienes. Swelling of the airway wall is caused by edema, with or without bronchoconstriction. Chronic inflammation can also lead to hypersecretion of mucus and exudation, resulting in plugging of the airways and, ultimately, matrix deposition and airway remodeling (see Figure 1.1).

Definition of asthma based on pathophysiology
Improved understanding of the inflammatory nature of asthma has led to an operational definition of the condition, in which

symptoms are related to the underlying pathophysiology (Table 1.2). Such a definition has important consequences for the diagnosis and treatment of asthma. Repeating lung function measurements to take account of the marked variation in airflow in asthma is an important element in the diagnosis (see Chapter 3). Similarly, recognition that asthma is a chronic inflammatory disorder has focused attention on the use of corticosteroids in the long-term management of the condition (see Chapter 4).

Risk factors for asthma

Asthma is a complex condition, and its causes are not fully understood. Risk factors can be classified as:

- host factors that predispose an individual to asthma
- causal factors, which are environmental factors that influence susceptibility to the development of asthma in predisposed individuals
- trigger factors, which are environmental factors that precipitate asthma exacerbations and/or cause symptoms to persist.

Examples of these factors are shown in Table 1.3. In any given individual, the development of asthma, and the occurrence of acute exacerbations, will be due to an interaction between numerous predisposing, environmental and occupational factors.

TABLE 1.2

An operational definition of asthma based on underlying pathophysiology

- Asthma is a chronic inflammatory disorder of the airways, in which many cells and cellular elements play a role

- The chronic inflammation causes an associated increase in airway hyperresponsiveness that leads to recurrent episodes of wheezing, breathlessness, chest tightness and cough, particularly at night and/or in the early morning

- Episodes of asthma symptoms are usually associated with widespread but variable airflow obstruction that is often reversible, either spontaneously or with treatment

TABLE 1.3

Potential risk factors for the development or exacerbation of asthma

Predisposing factors

- Genetic predisposition
- Atopy
- Airway hyperresponsiveness
- Sex
- Race/ethnicity

Causal factors

- Indoor allergens (domestic mites, animal allergens, cockroach allergen, fungi)
- Outdoor allergens (pollens, fungi)
- Occupational sensitizers
- Tobacco smoking (passive and active)
- Air pollution (outdoor and indoor)
- Respiratory infections
- Parasitic infections
- Socioeconomic status
- Family size
- Diet and drugs
- Obesity

Trigger factors

- Allergens
- Pollutants
- Respiratory infections
- Exercise and hyperventilation
- Changes in the weather
- Sulfur dioxide
- Foods, additives, drugs
- Extreme emotional expression
- Tobacco smoking
- Irritants (e.g. household sprays, paint fumes)

Predisposing factors. The most important factor predisposing to asthma is atopy. This is a condition characterized by excessive production of IgE in response to allergens. The prevalence of asthma increases with increasing serum IgE concentrations, and the majority of asthma patients (other than those developing the condition late in life) are atopic and, in particular, express IgE directed to inhaled allergens. Atopic diseases such as asthma tend to run in families, with heritability accounting for up to 50% of the clinical expression.

Childhood asthma is more common in boys than in girls until the age of about 10 years, when the difference disappears. Severe persistent asthma in adults is more frequent in women. There is some evidence that these differences are due to differences in allergen sensitivity and airway responsiveness between the sexes, although the differential effects of hormones at puberty may also lead to changes in asthma prevalence. Clearly, genetic influences can modify the risk of an individual developing atopy and asthma.

Hygiene hypothesis. A rise in the worldwide prevalence of asthma and allergic diseases has been documented in the past two decades, particularly in nations with a Western lifestyle. This rise has been particularly well described in Eastern European countries where the epidemiological findings of a rise in the prevalence of allergy and asthma have been associated with changes in lifestyle such as newer housing and increasing in-home childcare. In addition, a lower prevalence of asthma has been observed in children raised in a rural environment, suggesting that factors such as increased exposure to bacterial lipopolysaccharide, or altered gastrointestinal flora, may be associated with this trend.

The finding that childhood infections such as tuberculosis and hepatitis may be protective for allergy and asthma suggested the 'hygiene hypothesis', which attributes the rising prevalence of asthma and allergic diseases to a failure of early immune maturation caused by the relative protection from bacterial exposure in the first few years of life that a Western lifestyle offers. Lack of bacterial stimulation of the immature immune system is thought to skew the immune system to produce IgE in response to common allergens, rather than IgG.

More recently, it has been observed that other autoimmune diseases, such as juvenile diabetes mellitus and Crohn's disease, have also risen in prevalence. The hygiene hypothesis has therefore been modified to suggest that failure of bacterial immune stimulation early in life leads to altered maturation of immunoregulatory pathways through T-suppressor cells. Further understanding of

immune maturation is necessary before the networks involved can
be fully traced, but the hypothesis has lead to the identification of
some areas that show promise for the development of preventative
asthma interventions.

Causal factors. The most common causal factors for asthma are
inhaled allergens, especially those from indoor sources: domestic
mites, cats or dogs, and fungi. Outdoor pollens from grasses, trees
and wind-pollinated weeds are also common inhaled allergens.
Allergen exposure leads to the activation of specific T lymphocytes
and the production of specific IgE antibodies by B lymphocytes,
thereby sensitizing the individual to subsequent exposure. There is a
strong correlation between the prevalence of asthma and long-term
exposure to allergen, and asthma often improves when the allergen
is removed, although this is not always feasible.

Domestic mites appear to be the most common sources of indoor
allergens. The principal species involved are *Dermatophagoides
pteronyssinus, D. farinae, D. microceras* and *Euroglyphus mainei*,
which account for about 90% of mites in house dust in temperate
climates. The predominant allergens are cysteine and serine
proteases, and amylase, from the digestive tracts of the mites and
their feces. In inner cities and tropical environments, cockroaches
are also a source of asthmagenic allergens.

Domestic animals release allergens in their saliva, urine, feces and
danders. The most important allergen is the Fel d 1 allergen found
in cat fur and saliva. Allergic sensitivity to dogs is less common but,
nevertheless, up to 30% of allergic patients have positive skin tests
to dog allergens. Other domestic pets, particularly horses, rabbits,
guinea pigs, rats, gerbils and mice, are also important sources of
sensitizing allergen.

Both indoor and outdoor fungi can act as allergens. The most
important indoor fungi are *Penicillium, Aspergillus, Alternaria,
Cladosporium* and *Candida; Alternaria* and *Cladosporium* are also
outdoor allergens. Pollen allergens associated with asthma are
derived from trees (predominantly in early spring), grasses (late
spring and summer) and weeds (late summer and autumn).

In addition to allergens, occupational substances (Table 1.4), drugs and food additives can also produce airway sensitization and may play a causal role in up to 20% of individuals with asthma. High-molecular-weight sensitizers, such as grain, dust, urine and dander proteins from animals, probably cause sensitization by the same IgE-dependent mechanisms as allergens. The mechanism by which low-molecular-weight sensitizers (such as diisocyanates and platinum salts) act is unknown; however, there is increasing evidence that IgE plays a role here too. Among the most common causes of drug-induced asthma are aspirin and other non-steroidal anti-inflammatory drugs (NSAIDs), which trigger asthma attacks in between 4% and 28% of asthmatic patients in different countries. Intolerance to NSAIDs usually develops between 30 and 50 years of age, and persists throughout life. It may result from a defect in the oxidative metabolism of arachidonic acid, causing excessive production of a powerful class of bronchoconstricting mediators – the cysteinyl leukotrienes (cysLTs). Frequently, individuals with aspirin-intolerant asthma are not atopic, and may also have nasal polyposis.

Cigarette smoking is one of the potentially modifiable causes of asthma. Passive smoking in children exposed to cigarette smoke, especially from their mothers, is associated with a significantly increased risk of asthma and exacerbations. It is is also an important early-life risk factor for asthma, impairing lung growth and encouraging allergic responses in early infancy. In adults, there is some evidence that smoking may increase the risk of developing asthma after exposure to some occupational sensitizers. In addition, current smoking is associated with increased asthma symptoms and blunted response to preventive treatments, especially steroids.

Laboratory studies have identified a number of air pollutants as factors in worsening asthma, but epidemiological studies of the relationship between outdoor air pollution and asthma have yielded conflicting results. Although asthma is more common in industrialized countries (see Chapter 2), there is little evidence that air pollution alone is directly responsible for this increased prevalence. Similarly, indoor pollutants arising, for example, from

TABLE 1.4

Some causes of occupational asthma

Occupation/occupational field	Agent
	Animal proteins
Laboratory animal workers, vets	Dander and urine proteins
Food processing	Shellfish, egg proteins, pancreatic enzymes, amylase
Dairy farmers	Storage mites
Poultry farmers	Poultry mites, droppings, feathers
Granary workers	Storage mites, *Aspergillus*, indoor ragweed, grass
Research workers	Locusts
Fish-food manufacturing	Midges
Detergent manufacturing	*Bacillus subtilis* enzymes
Silk workers	Silkworm moths and larvae
	Plant proteins
Bakers	Flour, amylase
Food processing	Coffee-bean dust, meat tenderizer (papain), tea
Farmers	Soybean dust
Shipping workers	Grain dust (mold, insects, grain)
Laxative manufacturing	Ispaghula, psyllium
Sawmill workers, carpenters	Wood dust (western red cedar, oak, mahogany, zebrawood, redwood, Lebanon cedar, African maple, eastern white cedar)
Electric soldering	Colophony (pine resin)
Nurses	Psyllium, latex

(CONTINUED)

TABLE 1.4 (CONTINUED)

Some causes of occupational asthma

Occupation/occupational field	Agent
	Inorganic chemicals
Refinery workers	Platinum salts, vanadium salts
Plating	Nickel salts
Diamond polishing	Cobalt salts
Manufacturing	Aluminum fluoride
Beauticians	Persulfate
Welding	Stainless steel fumes, chromium salts
	Organic chemicals
Manufacturing	Antibiotics, piperazine, methyldopa, salbutamol, cimetidine
Hospital workers	Disinfectants (sulfathiazole, chloramine, formaldehyde, glutaraldehyde), latex
Anesthesiology	Enflurane
Poultry workers	Aprolium
Fur dyeing	Fur dye
Rubber processing	Formaldehyde, ethylene diamine, phthalic anhydride
Plastics industry	Toluene diisocyanate, hexamethyl diisocyanate, dephenylmethyl isocyanate, phthalic anhydride, triethylene tetramines, trimellitic anhydride, hexamethyl tetramine, acrylates
Automobile painting	Ethanolamine, diisocyanates
Foundry workers	Reaction product of furan binder

heating and cooking with gas, and organic chemicals used in buildings and furnishings, aggravate established asthma. However, these pollutants are not thought to contribute to the development of new asthma in individuals who otherwise would not have suffered from the condition.

The relationship between asthma and dietary factors is unclear. There is some evidence that asthma is associated with food allergy during infancy, which often precedes other atopic disorders such as allergic rhinitis and, frequently, asthma. Several trials of dietary modification to avoid highly 'allergenic' foods in pregnancy and in the first year of life have shown some benefit in delaying the onset of allergic diseases, but not in reducing the eventual occurrence of asthma. Therefore, dietary modifications during pregnancy and infancy to prevent asthma are not currently recommended. Exclusive breastfeeding for the first 6 months of life is supported. Epidemiological evidence suggests that diets high in fish oils, containing omega–3 fatty acids, may be protective against asthma, as may diets high in fruit and vegetables. However, these findings await confirmation from large prospective controlled trials.

Trigger factors can induce asthma by causing inflammation, provoking bronchial hyperresponsiveness, or both. Individual triggers vary markedly, and may also alter with time in the same patient. Common triggers include allergens, air pollutants, viral infections, exercise and hyperventilation, and emotional stress. In addition, adverse weather conditions have been associated with asthma exacerbations, but the relationship between asthma and climatic conditions has not been studied in detail.

Key points – pathophysiology

- Asthma is a chronic inflammatory condition of the conducting airways. It is characterized by recurrent episodes of airflow limitation, which, depending on the severity of the attack, can cause breathlessness, wheezing, chest tightness and cough.
- Structural changes also occur that are particularly evident in those with severe and chronic disease.
- A number of risk factors contribute to asthma, but the most prominent are allergen exposure in genetically susceptible subjects and maternal cigarette smoking.
- Genetic factors determine susceptibility to the environmental factors, and it is the interaction between these that leads to clinical disease.

Key references

Arshad SH. Primary prevention of asthma and allergy. *J Allergy Clin Immunol* 2005;116:3–14.

Bierman CW, Pealman DS, Shapiro GG, Busse WW, eds. *Allergy, Asthma and Immunology from Infancy to Adulthood*, 3rd edn. Philadelphia: WB Saunders, 1996.

Frew AJ, Bradding P, Johnston SL et al. Allergy. In: Tomlinson S, Heagerty AM, Weetman AP, eds. *Mechanisms of Disease: an Introduction to Clinical Science*. Cambridge: Cambridge University Press, 1997:129–59.

Holgate ST. The cellular and mediator basis of asthma in relation to natural history. *Lancet* 1997; 350(suppl II):5–9.

National Heart, Lung, and Blood Institute at the National Institutes of Health, and the World Health Organization. *GINA Workshop Report, Global Strategy for Asthma Management and Prevention*. Bethesda:NIH/NHLBI, 2002 (publication number 02-3659).

Schaub B, Lauener R, von Mutius E. The many faces of the hygiene hypothesis. *J Allergy Clin Immunol* 2006;117:969–77.

Asthma is one of the most common chronic diseases worldwide, but reliable epidemiological data are hard to obtain. The reported prevalence depends on the definition of asthma used, the age and socioeconomic status of the population studied, and the study design.

Prevalence

The prevalence of asthma in children varies from almost 0 to over 35% (Figures 2.1 and 2.2); in general, the highest prevalence is seen in affluent, westernized populations. In adults, prevalence estimates vary from less than 1% to 13%.

Within a particular country, the prevalence of asthma may differ markedly between different racial or ethnic groups. In the USA, for example, asthma is more common among black African-Americans than whites, but the difference is less pronounced in the UK. In the UK, the prevalence among Asians is lower than among whites.

Although reliable data are hard to obtain, studies have consistently shown that the prevalence of asthma increased worldwide during the 1990s (Figure 2.3). In many countries, numbers seem to have stabilized. The reasons for the increase in the prevalence of asthma are not clear, but may include:
- increased exposure to airborne allergens, particularly house-dust mites
- exposure to occupational allergens
- increased urbanization, and thus exposure to adjuvants such as certain respiratory viruses, dietary components and pollutants
- reduced exposure to bacterial and viral infections in early infancy.

Mortality and morbidity associated with asthma

Relatively few data are available on asthma mortality, and the existing data are difficult to interpret because of changes in

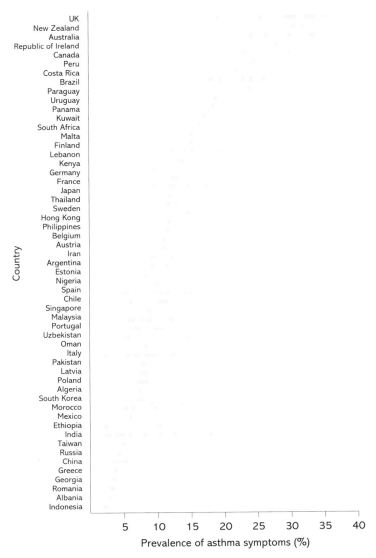

Figure 2.1 International and national variations in asthma prevalence suggest that environmental factors may affect asthma development in childhood. In the International Study of Asthma and Allergies in Childhood (ISAAC), children aged 13–14 years were asked to complete simple questionnaires about symptoms of asthma experienced in the past 12 months. Each dot represents the prevalence recorded at a particular center. Reproduced with permission from ISAAC Steering Committee 1998.

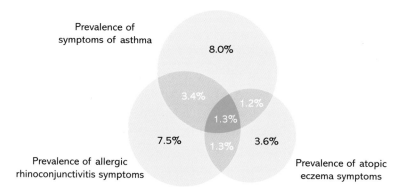

Figure 2.2 Overall proportion of children reporting symptoms of asthma and/or allergic rhinoconjunctivitis and/or atopic eczema in the previous 12 months in the International Study of Asthma and Allergies in Childhood (ISAAC). Reproduced with permission from ISAAC Steering Committee 1998.

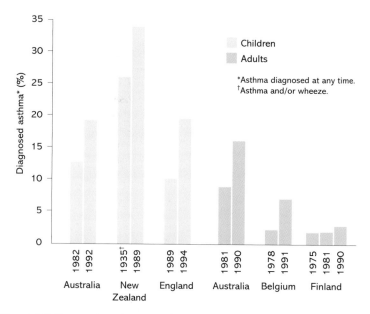

Figure 2.3 Changes in asthma prevalence with time in different countries. Data are taken from the National Heart, Lung, and Blood Institute at the National Institutes of Health, and the World Health Organization. *GINA Workshop Report, Global Strategy for Asthma Management and Prevention.* Bethesda:NIH/NHLBI, 2002 (publication number 02-3659).

diagnostic and reporting criteria during the past two decades. However, it appears that, for people under 35 years of age, reports of mortality due to asthma have an accuracy of over 85%. In older patients, the reported mortality due to asthma may be higher than the true figure, because some patients may have died from concomitant chronic obstructive pulmonary disease (COPD).

Mortality for patients of all ages in different countries between 1960 and 1990 is shown in Figure 2.4. In many countries, a marked increase in asthma deaths occurred in the 1960s, after which mortality tended to stabilize. In the UK, the mortality rate increased slightly during the 1980s, but the most recent data suggest that death rates are now falling. The greatest increase in mortality during the late 1970s and 1980s was seen in New Zealand (Figure 2.4). The reasons for this are unclear; the use of high doses of short-acting β_2-agonists, especially fenoterol, has been associated with the increased mortality, but the evidence is inconclusive. Ethnic

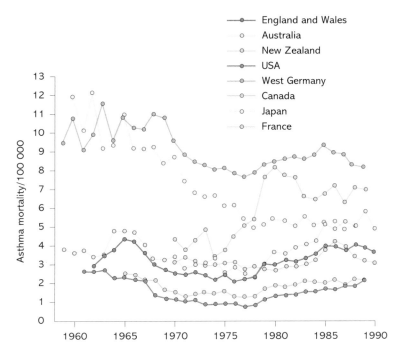

Figure 2.4 Deaths from asthma in patients of all ages, 1960–1990.

and socioeconomic factors may be at least partly responsible. In New Zealand, a large proportion of the increased mortality occurred in Maoris, and a similar increase occurred during the same period among black Americans living in inner-city areas of the USA. Studies of asthma deaths during this time suggested that a majority were preventable with best available current treatment, and that factors such as poor access to healthcare may have been partly responsible. In countries that have introduced effective guidelines for asthma management (e.g. the UK, Australia, Scandinavian countries), mortality is now declining.

In addition to being an important cause of death, asthma causes substantial morbidity and interference with everyday activities. Insights into the extent of asthma-related morbidity come from studies of hospital admission rates, which have shown that hospitalizations for asthma are increasing in a number of countries. Increasing morbidity may relate to a number of factors, including:

- the increasing prevalence of asthma
- increased exposure to trigger factors (e.g. allergens, pollutants, viruses)
- undertreatment with or reduced access to anti-inflammatory agents
- overdependence on bronchodilators
- failure to monitor lung function by regular PEF measurements
- delay in seeking medical attention during acute exacerbations.

In addition, in affluent countries, low income appears to be a risk factor for increased morbidity.

Early-life origins of asthma
Studies in neonates and young children born of allergic parents suggest that the atopic state begins to manifest itself very early in life. Thus, the findings of increased numbers of mast cells and eosinophils in the lavage fluid of children aged 3–5 years with asthma suggest that all the necessary cell and mediator pathways are already in place to express the full disease. Despite several recent large intervention studies, such as the Childhood Asthma Management Program (CAMP) and START (Inhaled Steroid

Treatment As Regular Therapy In Early Asthma), it is still not clear whether the introduction of inhaled corticosteroids early in life, at the onset of asthma, is able to influence the natural history of the disease or airway remodeling; two recent studies suggest that it does not.

There may be maternal risk factors that influence the genetic expression of allergy and asthma in the offspring. Several laboratories have now shown that lymphocytes present in the cord blood of babies of allergic mothers show delayed maturation, particularly in respect of the cytokine interferon-γ, which, under normal conditions, has the capacity to inhibit the development of the allergic pathways. The basis for this deficiency is far from clear, but it does provide one potential avenue for correcting an immunologic response early in life before the allergic cells are recruited into the lung.

Natural history of asthma

Asthma can occur at any time in life, although it most commonly develops in infancy and childhood. The natural history of the condition varies according to the age at onset, and possibly according to the causative factors.

Infancy. Asthma can develop during infancy, but it may be difficult to diagnose until the child is older. The most common cause of wheezing during the first months of life is viral respiratory infection. In some cases, wheezing during infancy may reflect small lung size, and will resolve with time; by contrast, wheezing due to asthma will persist into childhood.

In susceptible infants, atopy predisposes the airways to sensitization by allergens or environmental chemicals, resulting in recurrent wheezing. Wheezing and coughing may be infrequent, but in some children symptoms may have become common by an early age.

Childhood. Allergy, particularly to house-dust mite, is the most common feature associated with the development of asthma

Key points – epidemiology and natural history

- Asthma is one of the most common chronic diseases worldwide. The highest prevalence is seen in affluent, westernized populations.
- In many countries, asthma, along with other allergic disorders, continues to increase in prevalence, especially in children and young adults.
- In many countries, death from asthma reflects poor access to healthcare.
- Asthma can occur at any time in life, although it most commonly develops in infancy and childhood.
- There is evidence that early life events, including those that occur in the womb, may be important in the initiation of childhood asthma in those genetically at risk.
- Although asthma disappears in 30–50% of children during puberty, it often recurs in adulthood.
- There is no evidence that regular use of corticosteroids in early life alters the natural history of asthma, though they are highly effective in disease control.

during childhood. Viral infections are important triggers of exacerbations in children with atopic asthma, but there is little evidence that they are a direct cause of the development of asthma. By the age of 8 years, a significant proportion of children develop bronchial hyperresponsiveness and symptoms of moderate-to-severe asthma, whereas others continue to show mild intermittent asthma.

Lung growth is relatively normal in most children with mild asthma, but may be reduced in children with severe persistent symptoms. This is important because long-term studies show that, although asthma disappears in 30–50% of children during puberty, it often recurs in adulthood. Furthermore, lung function often remains impaired even when clinical signs of asthma have disappeared, and 5–10% of children with mild asthma develop severe asthma later in life. In general, children with mild asthma are likely to have a good prognosis, but those with moderate or severe asthma are likely to show some degree of bronchial hyperresponsiveness and to be at risk of the persistence of asthma throughout life.

There is no evidence that regular use of corticosteroids in early life alters the natural history of asthma, though they are highly effective in disease control.

Prevalence studies of asthma reveal that asthma is generally more common in boys until puberty, when more girls develop asthma and this predominance reverses. Many individuals acquire asthma in their adolescent years.

Adulthood. The development of asthma in adulthood is frequently associated with exposure to occupational sensitizers causing classic allergic responses or via mechanisms not involving IgE. It is not known what proportion of patients who develop asthma in adulthood actually had a history of childhood asthma; abnormal lung function or bronchial hyperresponsiveness persists in many patients whose symptoms disappear during childhood.

The natural history of late-onset asthma is variable. It appears that, in patients whose asthma develops after the age of about 50 years, lung function (as measured by the forced expiratory volume in 1 second, FEV_1) deteriorates at a faster rate than in those who develop asthma at an earlier age. Moreover, bronchial hyperresponsiveness appears to be associated with a faster rate of deterioration. Such older people with asthma have increasingly become the focus of attention as the mortality of this group is relatively high.

Key references

Holgate ST, ed. The rising trends in asthma. *Ciba Foundation Bull* 1997;206.

Holgate ST, Busse W, eds. *Asthma and Rhinitis: Implications for Diagnosis and Treatment*. Oxford: Blackwell Scientific Publications, 1995.

Holt PG, Upham JW, Sly PD. Contemporaneous maturation of immunologic and respiratory functions during early childhood: implications for development of asthma prevention strategies. *J Allergy Clin Immunol* 2005;116: 16–24.

International Study of Asthma and Allergies in Childhood (ISAAC) Steering Committee. Worldwide variation in prevalence of symptoms of asthma, allergic rhinoconjunctivitis, and atopic eczema: ISAAC. *Lancet* 1998;351: 1225–32.

National Heart, Lung, and Blood Institute at the National Institutes of Health, and the World Health Organization. *GINA Workshop Report, Global Strategy for Asthma Management and Prevention.* Bethesda: NIH/NHLBI, 2002 (publication number 02-3659).

Pauwels RA, Pedersen S, Busse W et al. Early intervention with budesonide in mild persistent asthma: a randomised controlled trial. *Lancet* 2003;361:1071–6.

Szefler S, Weiss S, Tonascia A et al. Long-term effects of budesonide or nedocromil in children with asthma. *N Engl J Med* 2000;343:1054–63.

Although asthma is one of the most common chronic disorders, it is often underdiagnosed, especially in older people. Because of the intermittent and non-specific nature of symptoms, patients may accept the effects of their condition and delay seeking treatment. They may also be incorrectly diagnosed when they do seek medical advice; in adults (particularly the elderly) and children, asthma is often misdiagnosed as bronchitis or 'wheezy' bronchitis and treated inappropriately with antibiotics. An accurate diagnosis is essential for effective asthma control.

Symptoms

The clinical diagnosis of asthma is often based on the presence of symptoms such as:

- breathlessness – often episodic
- wheezing
- chest tightness
- coughing.

These symptoms may be particularly marked at night and in the early hours of the morning.

The presence of symptoms, however, is not by itself sufficient for a diagnosis of asthma to be made; the history of symptoms and possible provocative factors must also be considered (Table 3.1), and the diagnosis confirmed by objective measures of lung function.

Various symptom scoring scales have been developed to monitor the occurrence and severity of symptoms. These can be useful in the management of individual patients, although it is important that they be adapted according to the patient's age and cultural background.

TABLE 3.1

Key questions to consider in making a diagnosis of asthma

A diagnosis of asthma should be considered if the answer to any of these questions is yes

- Has the patient had an attack or recurrent episodes of wheezing?
- Does the patient have a troublesome cough, particularly at night or on waking?
- Is the patient awoken by coughing or difficulty in breathing?
- Does the patient cough or wheeze after physical activity?
- Does the patient experience breathing difficulties during a particular season?
- Does the patient cough, wheeze or develop chest tightness after exposure to airborne allergens or irritants?
- Do colds go to the chest or take more than 10 days to resolve?
- Does the patient use any medication when symptoms occur? If so, how often?
- Are symptoms relieved when medication is used?

Physical examination

Asthma symptoms vary during the day, and the respiratory system may appear normal on physical examination. During asthma exacerbations, small airways are occluded because of a combination of bronchoconstriction, edema and hypersecretion of mucus. The patient therefore breathes at a higher lung volume to maintain airway patency; thus, clinical signs of dyspnea (Table 3.2) are more likely to be present during symptomatic exacerbations or if patients are examined in the morning before administration of a bronchodilator.

The absence of wheezing is not sufficient to preclude a diagnosis of asthma. In an exacerbation, some patients may have such severe obstruction of the airways that wheezing may not be noticeable. Such patients, however, usually have other signs of respiratory obstruction, such as difficulty in speaking, cyanosis, drowsiness and chest hyperinflation.

TABLE 3.2

Clinical signs of asthma

- Dyspnea
  - wheezing, particularly on expiration
  - use of the accessory muscles of respiration
  - flaring of the nostrils during inspiration (particularly in children)
  - interrupted talking
  - hyperinflation (use of accessory muscles, hunched shoulders, hunching forward or preferring not to lie down)
- Cough
  - chronic or recurring
  - worse at night and in the early hours of the morning; sleep disrupted
- Tachycardia
- Associated conditions
  - eczema
  - rhinitis
  - sinusitis
  - hay fever
- Cyanosis – life-threatening!
- Drowsiness – life-threatening!

Measurements of lung function

Patients with asthma often have poor recognition of their symptoms and poor perception of symptom severity. Measurements of lung function provide an objective assessment of airflow limitation, and its variability and reversibility, and thus are valuable in the diagnosis and management of asthma. Measurements widely used in patients over 5 years of age are FEV_1, forced vital capacity (FVC) and PEF.

FEV_1 and FVC are measured by spirometry. To make these measurements, patients are taught to perform a forced expiration after a maximal inspiration, and the highest of at least three reproducible measurements is recorded. Predicted values, based on age, sex, race and height, are available and can be compared with the patient's measurements to aid interpretation. The ratio of FEV_1 to FVC provides a useful measure of airway obstruction. Forced expiration normally produces FEV_1/FVC ratios of more than 70% (or 85% in children); ratios below these figures suggest airway obstruction, and the lower the ratio, the more severe the obstruction.

Spirometers have become smaller and more portable, and, while spirometry is usually carried out in the hospital or specialist setting, it is increasingly available in an office setting, such as a general practice. If spirometry is used to monitor patients, it is critical that the tester is appropriately trained in conducting the test and in maintaining the equipment to ensure reproducibility and comparability of measurements. For asthma diagnosis, spirometry is usually assessed before and after the administration of an inhaled short-acting β_2-agonist: responsiveness of FEV_1 by 15% or 200 mL (whichever is the greater) is indicative of asthma.

Measurement of PEF by means of a peak flow meter provides a useful and practical alternative to spirometry. In most patients, there is a good correlation between PEF and FEV_1. Peak flow meters are small, convenient, inexpensive and suitable for home use. They can be therefore be used both for the diagnosis of asthma in the clinic (Table 3.3) and to monitor asthma in the home. This

TABLE 3.3

Diagnosis of asthma from peak expiratory flow (PEF) measurements

- PEF increases by more than 15% and at least 60 L/min 15–20 minutes after inhalation of a short-acting β_2-agonist (e.g. salbutamol or terbutaline)

- PEF varies by more than 20% between morning measurement on waking and measurement 12 hours later

- PEF decreases by more than 15% after 6 minutes of running or other exercise

is important because, during acute exacerbations in some individuals, changes in PEF can precede the onset of symptoms; thus, early detection of such changes can allow appropriate treatment to be given. PEF readings can also indicate to an individual the severity of their asthma when compared with previous readings, enabling institution of a self-management plan.

Several types of peak flow meter are available, but the basic technique for use is the same in each case (Figure 3.1). Ideally, patients should measure PEF immediately on waking, before taking any bronchodilator medication, and last thing at night, after taking bronchodilator. Variability in daily PEF can then be calculated as a percentage of the mean daily value:

$$\text{Daily variability (\%)} = \frac{\text{PEF}_{\text{evening}} - \text{PEF}_{\text{morning}}}{^1/_2 \, (\text{PEF}_{\text{evening}} + \text{PEF}_{\text{morning}})} \times 100$$

Daily variability of more than 20% is indicative of asthma.

Measurement of bronchial responsiveness

Measurement of bronchial responsiveness can be useful in the diagnosis of asthma, although there is some overlap between the range of values found in patients with asthma and in those with rhinitis or other causes of lower airway obstruction, such as COPD. The most usual tests are performed in a lung function laboratory and involve the patient inhaling incremental doses of a bronchoconstricting substance, such as histamine, methacholine, hypertonic saline, AMP or mannitol; the changes in airway caliber are then followed by spirometry. The responsiveness of the airways is usually defined as that dose (D) or concentration (C) of agonist that reduces the FEV_1 by 20% of the starting volume (i.e. PD_{20} or PC_{20}). A standardized exercise test is also useful, especially for children with suspected asthma.

Skin-prick tests

Skin-prick tests with allergens or detection of allergen-specific IgE in the circulation are the most common diagnostic tests for allergy. For the diagnosis of asthma, the results of such tests

Put the disposable mouthpiece on the peak flow meter.

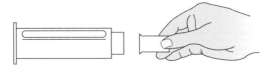

Stand up and hold the peak flow meter horizontally. Make sure that the end of the marker is at the end of the scale and that your hand is not restricting marker movement.

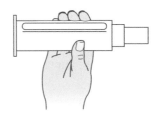

Breathe in as deeply as you can.

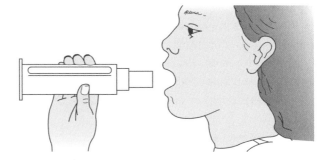

Then close your lips tightly around the mouthpiece and breathe out quickly. Note the results and repeat the procedure twice. Use the highest reading.

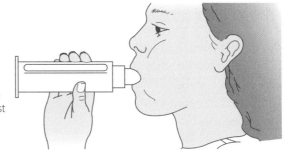

Figure 3.1 Use of a peak flow meter.

should always be interpreted in relation to the patient's history and the relationship between asthma symptoms and allergen exposure, because up to 40% of the population may exhibit atopy, but only a proportion of these individuals will have asthma. Nevertheless, the identification of allergens that may be contributing to persistent asthma and exacerbations is important in order to provide advice on allergen avoidance or other treatment strategies.

Patient groups

The diagnosis of asthma may be difficult in certain patient groups, especially smokers and the extremely young or old, who may have difficulty performing lung function tests.

Infants may have recurrent wheezing due to acute viral respiratory infections; the first episode of wheezing in infants under 6 months of age is usually due to viral bronchiolitis, whereas asthma is more likely to be the cause of wheezing after 18 months of age. After a viral infection symptoms may persist in children with atopic asthma. Similarly, older children may show asthma symptoms in association with viral infections or exercise; asthma should be considered if the child has a persistent nocturnal cough, or if colds go to the chest easily or take longer than 10 days to resolve.

Elderly patients. In older people, asthma may coexist with conditions such as COPD, bronchiectasis or interstitial pulmonary fibrosis. A history of asthma in childhood and variability on spirometry or PEF testing with β_2-agonists supports the diagnosis.

Occupational asthma is often misdiagnosed as chronic bronchitis or COPD. Ideally, diagnosis requires a detailed occupational history and the demonstration of a clear relationship between the development of symptoms at work and resolution of symptoms away from work.

Seasonal asthma associated with aero-allergens, such as the allergic rhinitis ('hay fever') suffered in the spring by pollen-sensitive individuals, may present as intermittent symptoms, with the patient being asymptomatic between seasons, or as seasonal worsening of moderate or severe asthma.

Cough-variant asthma. Patients present with cough as the principal symptom; they seldom wheeze. Coughing is often confined to the night, and examination during the day may not reveal evidence of abnormalities. Lung function tests and measurement of bronchial responsiveness with some form of challenge test are particularly important in such patients. Another helpful sign is eosinophils in the sputum (eosinophilic bronchitis).

Differential diagnosis

Wheezing can arise from either widespread or localized airway obstruction, and this should be considered in the differential diagnosis (Figure 3.2).

Breathlessness and cough are common symptoms of many conditions. The keys to diagnosing asthma are the patient's history

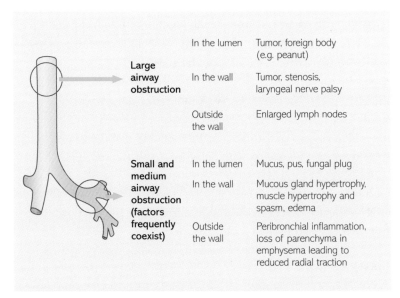

Figure 3.2 Differential diagnosis of obstructive airway disease. Reproduced with permission from Dr Martyn R Partridge.

Key points – diagnosis and classification

- Although asthma is one of the most common chronic disorders, it is often underdiagnosed.
- The clinical diagnosis of asthma is often based on the presence of symptoms, such as breathlessness (often episodic), wheezing, chest tightness and coughing.
- Objective measures of lung function are important in order to establish asthma as a diagnosis and to assess the response to treatment.
- Measurement of bronchial responsiveness and allergy status can aid diagnosis as well as identify possible preventative measures.
- Attempts should be made to assess disease severity to guide treatment.
- The diagnosis of asthma may be difficult in certain patient groups, especially those who smoke and the extremely young or old.

---

together with measurements of lung function through spirometry. An obstructive ventilatory defect suggests asthma or COPD while excluding other conditions. In adults, asthma-like symptoms can result from bronchitis or COPD; concomitant asthma and COPD are common among past or present smokers, and even occur in some individuals who have never smoked. Demonstration of reversible and variable airflow limitation confirms the diagnosis of asthma and indicates a trial of preventative treatment.

Although it is not always possible to distinguish asthma and COPD in those with a fixed component of airflow obstruction, detection of airflow obstruction does warrant a trial of therapy with inhaled corticosteroids to assess reversibility.

Classification of asthma severity

A combination of symptom measurements and lung function tests can be used to classify asthma according to its severity (Figure 3.3). These clinical measures of disease severity have been shown to

Step 4: severe persistent / continuous symptoms

Clinical features before treatment
- Continuous symptoms
- Frequent exacerbations
- Frequent nighttime asthma symptoms
- Physical activities limited by asthma symptoms
- Peak expiratory flow:
  - ≤ 60% predicted
  - variability > 30%

Daily medication required to maintain control
- Multiple daily controller (preventer) medications:
  - high-dose inhaled corticosteroid
  - long-acting bronchodilator
  - long-term oral corticosteroid

Step 3: moderate persistent

Clinical features before treatment
- Symptoms daily
- Exacerbations affect activity and sleep
- Nighttime asthma symptoms > once a week
- Daily use of inhaled short-acting β_2-agonist
- Peak expiratory flow or FEV_1:
  - > 60% – < 80% predicted
  - variability > 30%

Daily medication required to maintain control
- Daily controller (preventer) medications:
  - inhaled corticosteroid
  - long-acting bronchodilator (especially for nighttime symptoms)

Step 2: mild persistent

Clinical features before treatment
- Symptoms > once a week but < once a day
- Exacerbations may affect activity and sleep
- Nighttime asthma symptoms > twice a month
- Peak expiratory flow or FEV_1:
  - ≥ 80% predicted
  - variability 20–30%

Daily medication required to maintain control
- One daily controller (preventer) medication

FEV_1: forced expiratory volume in 1 second

Step 1: intermittent

Clinical features before treatment
- Intermittent symptoms < once a week
- Brief exacerbations (from a few hours to a few days)
- Nighttime asthma symptoms < twice a month
- Asymptomatic and normal lung function between exacerbations
- Peak expiratory flow:
  - ≥ 80% predicted
  - variability < 20%

Medication required to maintain control
- Intermittent reliever medication taken as needed only; inhaled short-acting β_2-agonist
- Intensity of treatment depends on severity of exacerbation: oral corticosteroids may be required

Figure 3.3 Classification of asthma severity. The presence of one of the features of severity is sufficient to place a patient in that category.

correlate well with pathological markers of airway inflammation, such as eosinophil numbers. Classification of asthma by severity is important because therapy takes a stepwise or graded approach in which the level of treatment increases with disease severity (see Chapter 4).

Patients often have a poor perception of the severity of their asthma, largely because they have adapted their lifestyle to accommodate their disease. There is also often a lack of lung function measurements to provide more objective information.

It is important to recognize that even mild asthma can be associated with severe, potentially fatal, exacerbations. Risk factors that have been shown to be associated with an increased risk of death from asthma include:

- a previous history of acute, life-threatening attacks
- hospitalization for asthma within the previous year
- psychosocial problems
- a history of intubation for asthma
- recent reduction or cessation of systemic corticosteroid therapy
- non-adherence to preventative treatments
- difficulty accessing treatment.

Conversely, a written asthma action plan has been found to be protective against asthma death.

Key references

Feather IH, Thompson PJ, Stewart GA et al. Cohabiting with domestic mites. *Thorax* 1993;48:5–9.

Hargreave FE. Investigation of airway inflammation in asthma: sputum examination. *Clin Exp Allergy* 1997;27(suppl 1):36–40.

Rusnak C, Bayram H, Devalia JL et al. Impact of the environment on allergic lung diseases. *Clin Exp Allergy* 1997;27(suppl 1):26–35.

Tinkelman DG, Naspitz CK, eds. *Childhood Asthma: Pathophysiology and Treatment,* 2nd edn. New York: Marcel Dekker, 1993.

The aims of asthma management are summarized in Table 4.1. Successful achievement of these aims requires attention to preventive measures (see Chapter 5), such as allergen avoidance, and the use of medication to prevent symptoms from developing and to treat acute attacks.

Drug classification

Drugs used in the management of asthma can be classified as controllers (also called preventers) or relievers.

- Controllers (preventers) are taken daily over the long term to control persistent asthma (Table 4.2). They include anti-inflammatory agents such as corticosteroids, sodium cromoglicate, nedocromil sodium and leukotriene modifiers, and long-acting bronchodilators such as long-acting β_2-agonists (LABAs) and sustained-release theophylline.

- Relievers (sometimes referred to as rescue medication) are used to reverse rapidly the bronchoconstriction and associated symptoms during acute attacks (Table 4.2). They include short-acting β_2-agonists, short-acting theophylline and short-

TABLE 4.1

Aims of asthma management

- Control of symptoms
- Prevention of exacerbations
- Maintenance of pulmonary function as close to normal levels as possible
- Maintenance of normal levels of activity
- Prevention of the development of irreversible airflow limitation
- Prevention of asthma mortality

TABLE 4.2

Effects of anti-asthma drugs, and risks of serious adverse events during long-term use

	Control of symptoms over weeks to months	Relief of exacerbations over minutes or hours	Risk of serious long-term adverse events
Inhaled corticosteroids	+++	–	+ (at high doses)
Oral corticosteroids (prednisolone)	++	++ (over hours)	+++
Sodium cromoglicate	+	–	–
Nedocromil sodium	+	–	–
Leukotriene modifiers	++	+	–
Short-acting inhaled β_2-agonists	+/–	+++	–
Long-acting inhaled β_2-agonists	++	++/+++	–
Oral β_2-agonists	+/–	++	+
Sustained-release theophylline	+	++	++
Inhaled anticholinergic agents	+	++	–

acting anticholinergic agents. The most effective forms are those that are delivered by inhalation directly to the airways.

Controller (preventer) medications

Inhaled corticosteroids, such as beclometasone dipropionate, budesonide, fluticasone propionate and ciclesonide, are the most effective anti-inflammatory agents currently available for asthma management. Studies have consistently shown that these agents reduce pathological signs of airway inflammation, so that lung function and symptoms improve, bronchial hyperresponsiveness decreases, and the frequency and severity of exacerbations is reduced. Corticosteroids act by interrupting the signaling pathways for proinflammatory molecules, by decreasing the expression of genes for a variety of inflammatory mediators, and by increasing the expression of genes for anti-inflammatory mediators.

Inhaled corticosteroids are also useful in the treatment of severe persistent asthma because they reduce the need for oral corticosteroids, and have fewer systemic adverse effects. Local adverse effects, which include oropharyngeal candidiasis, dysphonia and coughing, can largely be prevented by using spacer devices and mouth rinsing after use. Potential systemic adverse effects include thinning of the skin, cataract formation, adrenal suppression and decreased bone metabolism and growth. The risk of such effects depends on a number of factors, including the dose taken, absorption from the gut or lung, the extent of first-pass metabolism in the gut wall and liver, and the half-life of the corticosteroid. In general, the risk of significant systemic effects is low with therapeutic doses.

Systemic corticosteroids, such as prednisolone, can be given either orally or parenterally. Short courses (5–7 days) can be used when starting therapy in patients with uncontrolled asthma, or during periods of worsening asthma. Long-term treatment may be necessary in patients with severe persistent asthma; patients who require such medication should be seen by a specialist. Systemic events associated with oral corticosteroids include impairment of growth in children, osteoporosis, arterial hypertension, adrenal suppression, obesity, thinning of the skin, muscle weakness, cataract formation and diabetes. It should be noted that the safety of long-term inhaled corticosteroid therapy is better than that of oral or parenteral therapy.

Leukotriene modifiers. The cysteinyl leukotrienes (cysLTs) – LTC_4, LTD_4 and LTE_4 – are potent mediators of asthma. They are generated from arachidonic acid by the 5-lipoxygenase pathway that operates in mast cells and eosinophils. Once known as 'slow-reacting substance of anaphylaxis', cysLTs released during the inflammatory process cause prolonged contraction of smooth muscle, microvascular leaking and sputum secretion, and attract eosinophils. Since the structure of the leukotrienes was elucidated in 1979, a number of leukotriene-modifying drugs have been developed and introduced into the market. Zafirlukast, montelukast and pranlukast are new anti-asthma drugs that inhibit the effect of leukotrienes at their receptor (cysteinyl leukotriene receptor, cysLTR1). In addition, inhibitors of 5-lipoxygenase, such as zileuton, interrupt the conversion of arachidonic acid into leukotrienes, including the cysLTs and leukotriene B_4.

Treatment with one of these oral drugs can produce improvement in pulmonary function, protection from exercise-induced asthma and reduced eosinophilic inflammation. A clinical response is usually seen within 3 weeks of therapy, though not all patients benefit. Patients with asthma associated with intolerance to aspirin and other NSAIDs seem to be particularly responsive.

Leukotriene modifiers can be used to treat mild persistent asthma, especially in children, in whom concerns regarding effects on growth limit the use of inhaled corticosteroids, but are less effective overall than a low dose of inhaled corticosteroid. They can also be used together with an inhaled corticosteroid in moderate and severe asthma, but are less effective than the combination of an inhaled corticosteroid and an inhaled LABA. Clearly, the advantages of these drugs over other long-term controllers (preventers) are that they are orally administered and are not corticosteroids and, therefore, patient acceptability and adherence is likely to be good.

Sodium cromoglicate and nedocromil sodium. Inhaled sodium cromoglicate and nedocromil sodium inhibit allergen-induced airflow limitation and acute airflow limitation after exercise or exposure to cold air or sulfur dioxide. Each agent can be used as long-term therapy early in the course of asthma; a 4–6 week course may be needed to determine efficacy in a given patient. Adverse effects are few, although coughing may result from inhalation of the powder formulation. The mechanisms of action are not fully understood, but may involve a combination of inhibition of IgE-dependent mediator release, and blockade of sensory nerve pathways. Both agents can be used as maintenance therapy for asthma but are less effective than a low dose of inhaled corticosteroids.

Sustained-release theophylline. Theophylline is a bronchodilator, and there is some evidence that it may also have anti-inflammatory effects. It is both an inhibitor of cyclic AMP phosphodiesterase and an antagonist of adenosine receptors. During long-term treatment, sustained-release theophylline controls symptoms and improves lung function. Because of its long duration of action, it is useful in controlling nocturnal symptoms that persist despite regular anti-inflammatory treatment. However, theophylline has a number of potentially serious adverse effects (Table 4.3), and theophylline intoxication can result in seizures and death. Furthermore, the drug has a relatively narrow therapeutic index; serum concentrations producing adverse effects are close to those required for therapeutic efficacy. Appropriate dosing and monitoring are therefore essential; in general, dosing should produce a steady-state serum theophylline

TABLE 4.3

Adverse effects associated with theophylline

- Nausea
- Vomiting
- Gastrointestinal disturbances
- Tachycardia
- Palpitations
- Arrhythmias
- Headache
- Insomnia
- Convulsions

concentration of 5–15 µg/mL. Monitoring is advisable when treatment is started and at regular intervals thereafter. In addition, serum drug concentrations should be monitored if:

- adverse events occur with the usual dose
- the expected therapeutic benefit is not achieved
- the patient has a condition that is likely to affect theophylline metabolism (e.g. febrile illness, pregnancy, liver disease, congestive heart failure)
- the patient is receiving concomitant treatment with drugs that interact with theophylline (e.g. cimetidine, some quinolone antibiotics).

Long-acting β_2-agonists (LABAs), such as salmeterol and formoterol, have a duration of action of more than 12 hours. They act by relaxing airway smooth muscle, enhancing mucociliary clearance, and decreasing vascular permeability; in addition, they may modulate mediator release from mast cells and basophils. Long-term treatment with inhaled preparations improves symptoms and lung function, relieves nocturnal asthma and reduces the need for short-acting β_2-agonists. Such preparations can be used in patients for whom standard starting doses of inhaled corticosteroids do not control symptoms, as a more effective alternative to increasing the corticosteroid dose. LABAs should not be given without an inhaled corticosteroid.

Oral preparations are also available; these may be useful in controlling nocturnal symptoms when standard doses of inhaled corticosteroids, sodium cromoglicate or nedocromil sodium are ineffective.

Adverse events associated with LABAs include cardiovascular stimulation, anxiety, heartburn and tremor. The risk of systemic adverse effects is lower with inhaled therapy than with oral preparations.

Combination therapy. A series of clinical trials has shown that the inhaled LABAs salmeterol and formoterol, when administered to patients who are already taking inhaled corticosteroids but whose asthma is poorly controlled, may produce greater improvements in pulmonary function and symptom control than would be obtained by doubling the dose of inhaled corticosteroid. Combinations of a LABA and an inhaled corticosteroid are now available in single inhalers. It would seem, therefore, that the dose–response curve for topical corticosteroids is not linear, and that the overall benefits obtained with doses of up to approximately 800 µg beclometasone dipropionate per day are as great as those that can be achieved with further increments. One possible explanation for these observations is that topical corticosteroids are able to control the inflammatory response by inhibiting cytokine and other relevant pathways. They are not able to alter, at least in the short and medium term, the behavior of the remodeled airway with its increased smooth muscle, microvasculature and thickened airway walls. In this situation, drugs that act on the airway smooth muscle and microvasculature to restore airway physiology to normal are likely to be effective.

Reliever medications

Short-acting β_2-agonists. Inhaled short-acting β_2-agonists, such as salbutamol and terbutaline, are used to control bronchoconstriction, and are the treatment of choice for the management of acute exacerbations and the prophylaxis of exercise-induced asthma. Oral preparations are also available, and are suitable for patients who are unable to use inhaled medication.

Concern has been expressed over the long-term safety of the repeated use of the inhaled short-acting β_2-bronchodilators. Several points are worth making in relation to the use of these quick relievers. They are certainly the best drugs for relieving acute bronchospasm, but their increased use by a patient is a sign of worsening of asthma and the need for greater use of controller (preventer) drugs. The use of one canister of a metered-dose inhaler per month should certainly sound alarm bells. Regular use of short-acting β_2-agonists is not recommended, as a refractory response may develop, and it has been suggested that asthma may worsen. In addition, it is now known that genetic β_2-adrenoceptor polymorphisms dictate the effectiveness of these drugs, particularly with regard to tachyphylaxis or the development of refractoriness; therefore short-acting β_2-agonists should only be used for quick relief on an 'as-required' basis.

Systemic corticosteroids. Oral corticosteroid preparations have a relatively slow onset of action (4–6 hours), but may be useful in the treatment of severe acute exacerbations because they prevent progression of the exacerbation. As a result, they also reduce the need for emergency treatment or hospitalization, prevent early relapse and reduce the morbidity associated with exacerbations. Treatment is normally continued for 3–10 days after the exacerbation; the dose can be reduced and stopped as symptoms resolve and lung function returns to the personal best level.

Anticholinergic agents. Inhaled anticholinergic agents, such as ipratropium bromide or oxitropium bromide, cause bronchodilatation by inhibiting postganglionic efferent vagal fibers, thereby reducing the vagal tone on the airways. They also inhibit reflex bronchoconstriction provoked by inhaled irritants. They are less effective than inhaled β_2-agonists and have a slower onset of action, taking 30–60 minutes to reach their maximum effect. They are particularly useful in acute severe asthma exacerbations and as long-term therapy for patients with COPD. Adverse effects include dry mouth and a bad taste.

Short-acting theophylline. Oral treatment with short-acting theophylline has been used for pretreatment of exercise-induced asthma and for symptomatic relief. The role of theophylline in the treatment of exacerbations is controversial and it is now rarely used in developed countries, except for acute, severe, life-threatening asthma, because of the high risk of adverse effects and the slow onset of action.

Delivery of inhaled medication
Drug delivery by inhalation of aerosols or powders has the advantages of achieving high drug concentrations in the airways

and reducing the risk of systemic adverse effects. A variety of delivery devices are available (Table 4.4). Whichever device is chosen, its use should be explained carefully to the patient (Figures 4.1 and 4.2), and the patient's technique checked regularly.

Pressurized metered-dose inhalers (pMDIs) have, hitherto, been the most widely used types of inhaler, but their use is declining in many countries because of concern about the environmental effects of chlorofluorocarbons (CFCs) used as propellants. They deliver a measured dose of medication, and delivery is efficient when the device is used correctly (Figure 4.1).

Many patients, however, are unable to coordinate inspiration with inhaler actuation. The use of a spacer device (Figures 4.3 and 4.4) can overcome this problem to some extent. The medication is discharged into the spacer and held in suspension for several seconds. During this time, the patient can inhale the drug in one or several breaths, without the need to coordinate inspiration and drug delivery; this may be particularly useful in small children and patients with poor coordination. A small-volume spacer can be adapted with a face mask for young children.

In addition, the use of spacers reduces oropharyngeal deposition of drug and the incidence of local side effects, and allows high doses to be given during attacks.

Inhalers containing 'ozone-friendly' propellants, such as hydrofluoroalkanes, have been introduced to replace the CFC-

TABLE 4.4

Devices for delivery of aerosolized medication in asthma

- Pressurized metered-dose inhalers (pMDIs)
- Breath-actuated pMDIs (e.g. Autohaler)
- Dry-powder inhalers (DPIs) such as Accuhaler, Diskhaler, Rotahaler, Spinhaler and Turbohaler
- Spacer devices (e.g. AeroChamber, Babyhaler, Nebuhaler, Volumatic)
- Nebulizers

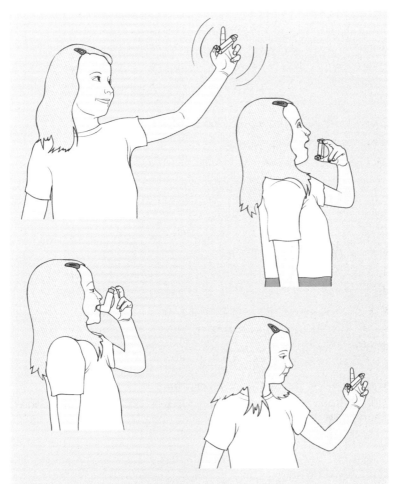

Pressurized metered-dose inhaler – instructions for use

- Shake the inhaler and take off the cap
- Stand up and breathe out
- Hold the mouthpiece in your mouth or just in front
- Breathe in slowly and deeply while pressing the canister down
- Hold your breath for 10 seconds
- Breathe out
- Wait for 30 seconds before repeating

Figure 4.1 Technique for use of a metered-dose inhaler without a spacer device.

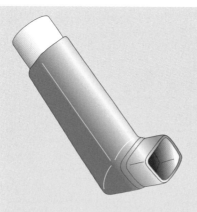

Pressurized metered-dose inhaler
(Detailed instructions for use are given in Figure 4.1)

Turbohaler – instructions for use

- Hold Turbohaler upright and twist blue grip forwards and backwards
- Breathe out gently
- Put mouthpiece between lips and breathe in deeply
- Remove inhaler and hold your breath for 10 seconds

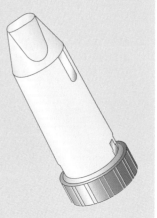

Autohaler – instructions for use

- Push the lever up and shake the inhaler
- Breathe out gently
- Put mouthpiece in mouth; ensure that the air vents at the bottom of the inhaler are not blocked
- Breathe in steadily; continue after the inhaler clicks
- Hold your breath for 10 seconds
- Lower lever on inhaler
- Wait at least 60 seconds before taking the next inhalation

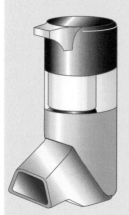

Figure 4.2 Different inhaler devices and instructions for their use.

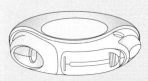

Accuhaler (Diskus) – instructions for use

- Hold the outer casing in one hand while pushing the thumb grip away until you hear a click

- With the mouthpiece towards you, slide the lever away until it clicks; this makes the dose available and moves the counter on

- Breathe out gently away from mouthpiece, then put mouthpiece in mouth and breathe in

- Remove inhaler and hold your breath for 10 seconds

- Close by sliding thumb grip back towards you until it clicks

Diskhaler – instructions for use

To load:

- Remove mouthpiece cover; pull the tray out gently until you can squeeze the ridges on each side and slide it out

- Place the foil disk on the wheel, numbers upwards, and slide the tray back

- Hold the corners of the tray and slide it in and out to rotate the disk until the highest number (8 or 4) shows in the window

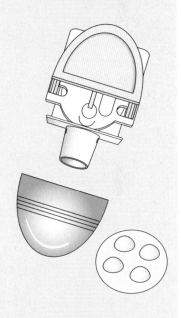

To use:

- Keeping the Diskhaler level, raise the rear of the lid as far as it will go so that the pin pierces the blister in the disk

- Still keeping the Diskhaler level, breathe out gently, put mouthpiece in mouth and breathe in as deeply as possible; do not block the two small air vents on the sides of the mouthpiece

- Remove Diskhaler from mouth and hold your breath for 10 seconds

- Slide tray in and out to prepare next dose

(a)   **(b)**

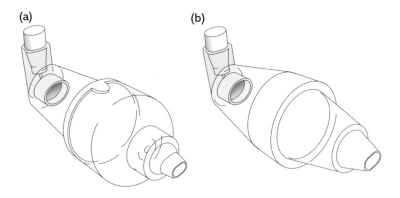

Figure 4.3 Spacer devices for use by (a) young children who need assistance and (b) patients who can use the device without help.

(a) Spacer device – instructions for parents/carers

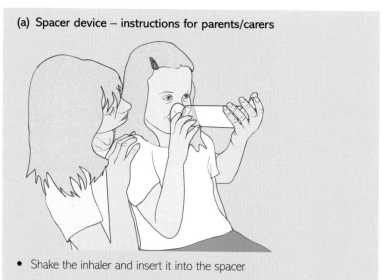

- Shake the inhaler and insert it into the spacer
- Put the mouthpiece into the child's mouth and seal the child's lips around the mouthpiece
- The child should breathe in and out slowly and gently
- Depress the canister as the child continues to breathe in and out several more times
- Remove the spacer from the child's mouth

Figure 4.4 (a) Use of a spacer by a young child.

containing pMDIs. Dissolution of the topical corticosteroid beclometasone dipropionate in a hydrofluoroalkane leads to the release of smaller particles on activation of the inhaler, and thus improved drug deposition and efficacy, but at the expense of greater systemic bioavailability from lung absorption and, therefore, an increased risk of side effects, unless the dose is adjusted accordingly.

Breath-actuated inhalers. These devices, in which the valve is actuated during inspiration, are useful in patients who have difficulty coordinating actuation and breathing. Drug deposition

(b) Spacer device – instructions for people who need no help

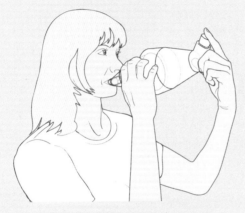

- Shake inhaler and insert it into the spacer
- Put the mouthpiece in your mouth
- Press the canister and breathe in slowly and deeply
- Hold your breath for 10 seconds*
- Breathe out through the mouthpiece
- Breathe in again, but do not press the canister this time
- Remove the device and wait for 30 seconds before taking another inhalation

   *Alternatively, breathe normally through the spacer for at least four breaths.

Figure 4.4 (b) Use of a spacer by a patient who can operate it without help.

appears to be greater than with pMDIs. As with pMDIs, however, propellants are needed to discharge the drug.

Dry-powder inhalers (DPIs) require a different inhalation technique from pMDIs. No propellant is needed because the drug is released by inspiratory airflow. However, a certain minimum flow rate is required, and thus these devices may be less effective in young children and during severe attacks. Inhalation of dry particles can cause coughing.

Nebulizers generate a wet aerosol by blowing compressed air through a drug solution or suspension, or by ultrasonic vibration. The patient inhales the aerosol through a face mask or mouthpiece. In most circumstances, nebulizers have been replaced in emergency settings, and for young children, by pMDIs and spacers, which have been demonstrated to provide equivalent drug delivery. This removes the need to purchase a nebulizer and air pump, and the problems of portability of this equipment in emergency or remote settings. Nebulized therapy is still used for those with very severe lung disease or extreme attacks. A standard dose of nebulized β_2-agonist is equivalent to 12–16 puffs from a pMDI and spacer.

Stepwise approach to asthma treatment

Current management guidelines recommend a stepwise approach to asthma treatment, depending on disease severity (see Figure 3.3), in both adults (Figure 4.5) and children (Figure 4.6). Four steps are recognized, depending on whether asthma is intermittent, mild persistent, moderate persistent or severe persistent. Patients should be started on the regimen most appropriate to the initial severity of their condition, and treatment stepped up or down according to the response. It should be noted that the management plans shown in Figures 4.5 and 4.6 are suggestions only; specific plans should be developed to meet the needs of individual patients (see Chapter 5). For example, some physicians like to control asthma by using a short course of oral corticosteroids, or a higher dose of inhaled corticosteroids, which can be reduced to a maintenance level once

Step 4: severe persistent / continuous symptoms

Controller (preventer)
Daily medications
- Inhaled corticosteroid (BDP > 1000 µg or equivalent) *plus* long-acting inhaled β_2-agonist *plus* one or more of the following if needed:
  - sustained-release theophylline
  - leukotriene modifier
  - long-acting oral β_2-agonist
  - oral corticosteroid

Reliever
- Short-acting bronchodilator: inhaled β_2-agonist as needed for symptoms

Avoid or control triggers

Step 3: moderate persistent

Controller (preventer)
Daily medications
- Inhaled corticosteroid (BDP 200–1000 µg or equivalent) *plus* long-acting inhaled β_2-agonist
Other options
- Inhaled corticosteroid (BDP 500–1000 µg or equivalent) *plus* sustained-release theophylline
- Inhaled corticosteroid (BDP 500–1000 µg or equivalent) *plus* long-acting oral β_2-agonist
- Inhaled corticosteroid at higher doses (BDP > 1000 µg or equivalent)
- Inhaled corticosteroid (BDP 500–1000 µg or equivalent) *plus* leukotriene modifier

Reliever
- Short-acting bronchodilator: inhaled β_2-agonist as needed for symptoms, not to exceed 3–4 times in one day

Step down
Review treatment every 3–6 months. If control is sustained for at least 3 months, a gradual stepwise reduction in treatment may be possible

Avoid or control triggers

Step 2: mild persistent

Controller (preventer)
Daily medication
- Inhaled corticosteroid (BDP ≤ 500 µg or equivalent)
Other options
- Sustained-release theophylline
- Cromones
- Leukotriene modifier

Reliever
- Short-acting bronchodilator: inhaled β_2-agonist as needed for symptoms, not to exceed 3–4 times in one day

Avoid or control triggers

Step 1: intermittent

Controller (preventer)
- None needed

Reliever
- Short-acting bronchodilator: inhaled β_2-agonist as needed for symptoms but less than once a week
- Intensity of treatment will depend on severity of attack
- Inhaled β_2-agonist or cromoglicate before exercise or exposure to allergen

Step up
If control is not achieved, consider step up. But first: review patient medication technique, adherence and environmental control (avoidance of allergens or other trigger factors)

Avoid or control triggers

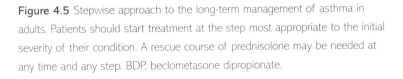

Figure 4.5 Stepwise approach to the long-term management of asthma in adults. Patients should start treatment at the step most appropriate to the initial severity of their condition. A rescue course of prednisolone may be needed at any time and any step. BDP, beclometasone dipropionate.

Step 4: severe persistent / continuous symptoms

Controller (preventer)
Daily medication
- Inhaled corticosteroid (budesonide > 800 µg or equivalent) *plus* one or more of the following if needed:
  - long-acting inhaled β_2-agonist
  - leukotriene modifier
  - sustained-release theophylline
  - oral corticosteroid

Reliever
- Inhaled short-acting bronchodilator: inhaled β_2-agonist *or*
- β_2-agonist tablets or syrup as needed for symptoms, not to exceed 3–4 times in one day

Avoid or control triggers

Step 3: moderate persistent

Controller (preventer)
Daily medication
- Inhaled corticosteroid (budesonide 200–400 µg) *plus* long-acting inhaled β_2-agonist
Other options
- Inhaled corticosteroid 500–800 µg *plus* leukotriene modifier
- Inhaled corticosteroid 500–800 µg *plus* long-acting oral β_2-agonist
- Inhaled corticosteroid at higher doses (> 1000 µg)
- Inhaled corticosteroid 500–800 µg *plus* sustained-release theophylline

Reliever
- Inhaled short-acting bronchodilator: inhaled β_2-agonist *or*
- β_2-agonist tablets or syrup as needed for symptoms, not to exceed 3–4 times in one day

Step down
Review treatment every 3–6 months. If control is sustained for at least 3 months, a gradual stepwise reduction in treatment may be possible

Avoid or control triggers

Step 2: mild persistent

Controller (preventer)
Daily medication
- Inhaled corticosteroid (budesonide 100–200 µg or equivalent)
Other options
- Cromones
- Leukotriene modifier
- Sustained-release theophylline

Reliever
- Inhaled short-acting bronchodilator: inhaled β_2-agonist *or*
- β_2-agonist tablets or syrup as needed for symptoms, not to exceed 3–4 times in one day

Avoid or control triggers

Step 1: intermittent

Controller (preventer)
- None needed

Reliever
- Inhaled short-acting bronchodilator: inhaled β_2-agonist
- Intensity of treatment will depend on severity of attack

Step up
If control is not achieved, consider step up. But first: review patient medication technique, adherence and environmental control (avoidance of allergens or other trigger factors)

Avoid or control triggers

Figure 4.6 Stepwise approach to the long-term management of asthma in children. Patients should start treatment at the step most appropriate to the initial severity of their condition. A rescue course of prednisolone may be needed at any time and any step.

clinical remission has been induced. This latter approach is one of the alternatives advocated in the British Thoracic Society/Scottish Intercollegiate Guidelines Network *British Guideline on the Management of Asthma*.

Step 1: intermittent asthma. Asthma is classified as intermittent if:
- symptoms occur less than once a week over a 3-month period
- exacerbations are brief, lasting from a few hours to a few days
- nocturnal symptoms do not occur more than twice a month
- the patient is asymptomatic between exacerbations and lung function is normal (PEF at or above 80% of predicted best with less than 20% variability).

Controller (preventer) medication is not needed in patients with intermittent asthma; inhaled bronchodilators (preferably short-acting β_2-agonists) are used as required to treat symptoms, but should be used less than once a week. The intensity of treatment of exacerbations will depend on the severity of the exacerbation (Table 4.5).

Step 2: mild persistent asthma. Patients are regarded as having mild persistent asthma if they experience exacerbations, persistent symptoms or persistent deterioration in lung function sufficiently often to warrant daily long-term treatment with controller (preventer) medication; for example, symptoms at least once a week but less than once a day over the previous 3 months, or chronic symptoms requiring treatment almost every day and nocturnal asthma more than twice a month.

Baseline PEF in patients with mild persistent asthma is equal to or greater than 80% of predicted, and PEF variability is 20–30%. Such patients require daily controller medication with anti-inflammatory agents. The recommended treatment is a low dose of inhaled corticosteroid. Other treatment options are sodium cromoglicate, nedocromil sodium, sustained-release theophylline or leukotriene modifiers. Patients should also be given reliever therapy (preferably a short-acting β_2-agonist) to be used as needed.

TABLE 4.5

Classification of severity of asthma exacerbations

	Mild	Moderate
Breathless	When walking	When talking Infants: softer, shorter cry, difficulty feeding Can lie down
Speech: talks in...	Sentences	Phrases
Alertness	May be agitated	Usually agitated
Respiratory rate*	Increased	Increased
Accessory muscles and suprasternal retractions	Usually not	Usually
Wheeze	Moderate, often only end-expiratory	Loud
Pulse†	< 100 beats/minute	100–200 beats/minute
Pulsus paradoxus	Absent (< 10 mmHg)	May be present (unreliable) (10–25 mmHg)
PEF after bronchodilator (% predicted or personal best)	> 80%	Approximately 60–80%
PaO_2 (on air)	Normal; test not usually necessary	> 60 mmHg
and/or $PaCO_2$	< 45 mmHg	< 45 mmHg
SaO_2 (on air)	> 95%	91–95%

Not all features may be present in any one exacerbation

*Normal rates in children: < 2 months, 60 breaths/minute; 2–12 months, < 50 breaths/minute; 1–5 years, < 40 breaths/minute; 6–8 years, < 30 breaths/minute

†Normal rates in children: 2–12 months, < 160 beats/minute; 1 year, < 120 beats/minute; 2–8 years, < 110 beats/minute

PEF, peak expiratory flow; PaO_2, partial pressure of oxygen in arterial blood; $PaCO_2$, partial pressure of carbon dioxide in arterial blood; SaO_2, oxygen saturation in arterial blood

Review proofs only: not for reproduction. Property of Health Press Limited.

Severe	Respiratory arrest imminent
At rest Infants: stops feeding	
Prefers sitting	Hunched forwards
Words	
Usually agitated	Drowsy or confused
Often > 30 breaths/minute	
Usually	Paradoxical thoraco- abdominal movement
Usually loud	Absent
> 120 beats/minute	Bradycardia
Often present (> 25 mmHg in adults, 20–40 mmHg in children)	Absence suggests respiratory muscle fatigue
< 60% (< 200 liters/minute in adults), or bronchodilator response lasts < 2 hours	
< 60 mmHg; possible cyanosis	
> 45 mmHg; possible respiratory failure	
< 90%	

Step 3: moderate persistent asthma is characterized by:
- daily symptoms over a prolonged period, or nocturnal asthma more than once a week
- a baseline PEF between 60% and 80% of predicted
- PEF variability of greater than 30%.

Control of moderate persistent asthma may require higher doses of inhaled corticosteroids than mild asthma; a long-acting inhaled β_2-agonist should be added to the inhaled corticosteroid. Other treatment options include the combination of inhaled corticosteroids and slow-release theophylline or a leukotriene modifier. The approach to symptomatic relief is the same as for mild persistent asthma. Oral corticosteroids may, however, be needed to control severe exacerbations.

Step 4: severe persistent asthma is characterized by:
- continuous, highly variable symptoms
- frequent nocturnal symptoms
- limitation of activity
- severe exacerbations despite medication
- baseline PEF less than or equal to 60% of predicted
- PEF variability greater than 30%.

Control of asthma may not be possible in this situation, and the aim of treatment is to achieve the best possible results in terms of symptom relief, increased airflow and reduced need for rescue medication. Treatment usually requires multiple daily administration of controller (preventer) medication, including high doses of inhaled corticosteroids and long-acting bronchodilators.

The decision to move to the next step should not be made until it has been confirmed that the patient's inhaler technique is satisfactory, that he or she has access to and is taking the treatment, and adequate allergen or irritant avoidance measures are being used. Once control has been achieved, treatment should be reviewed every 3–6 months; it may be possible to move the patient gradually to a lower step if control is maintained for at least 3 months.

Stepwise treatment in infants and young children. The basic
principles of this approach are similar to those for older patients.
However, only inhaled corticosteroids have been shown to be
effective as controller (preventer) medications in children under
3 years of age; long-acting inhaled β_2-agonists are less effective
in children than in adults. Sustained-release theophylline should
only be used if serum drug levels are monitored, because infants
with frequent febrile illnesses are at high risk of adverse effects.
Inhaled medication can be given by a pMDI with a spacer and
valve system, a face mask (for those under 4 years of age) or
a nebulizer.

Management of an acute asthma attack

Patients at risk. All patients with asthma, of any severity, can
suffer from an acute asthma episode, often described as an
asthma attack. The most common reason for an asthma attack is
viral respiratory infections, which are responsible for over 50%
of hospital admissions for asthma in adults. Such infections can
be responsible for a rapid decline in lung function, which may not
be entirely prevented by regular inhaled controller (preventer)
therapy.

   Other causes of acute asthma include acute allergen exposure,
when an allergic person is exposed to an allergen not usually
encountered in the environment. 'Thunderstorm asthma' is a
specific example. Epidemics of asthma can occur in people who
usually have allergic rhinitis due to grass pollens if a thunderstorm
occurs in spring or summer, when grass pollens are in the air; the
pollen grains can burst in the storm, permitting the inhalation of
smaller pollen allergens into the lower respiratory tract and thus
causing an asthma attack. Similarly, severe food allergies, such as
may occur to peanuts or shellfish, may be involved. Individuals with
such a food allergy often present with signs of anaphylaxis, but for
some, acute asthma is a major component of a severe food reaction
and requires recognition and treatment in its own right.

   Some medications, such as β-blockers, even in eye drops, may
also be responsible for an acute exacerbation of asthma. Individuals

with aspirin-sensitive asthma may have severe asthma after taking aspirin or other NSAIDs. NSAID reactions are most often described in individuals with non-allergic asthma who have nasal polyposis. Individuals with this type of asthma must avoid aspirin and all NSAIDs.

Regular use of controller asthma medication substantially reduces, but does not completely eliminate, the risk of an acute asthma attack. Asthma exacerbations may occur in individuals with asthma who do not receive adequate controller treatment. All individuals who present with an acute exacerbation should be asked what controller treatment they are taking, and consideration should be given to introducing or adjusting regular maintenance medication in order to prevent such exacerbations in the future.

How to recognize a severe attack. It is important for both patients and clinicians to recognize the signs of a severe asthma attack, and to know when to seek further help.

Patients can recognize a severe asthma attack by the frequency and severity of symptoms (Figure 4.7). Asthma symptoms that recur and require bronchodilator treatment more frequently than once every 4 hours are an indication of an attack that requires medical treatment. Most often, patients with a severe exacerbation of asthma describe their asthma as being 'out of control'. This is a clear sign that urgent help is needed. Patients may also monitor their PEF. A measurement of 50% of predicted or less that does not respond promptly to bronchodilator treatment is an indication for seeking emergency help.

Clinicians should assess the severity of an acute attack of asthma according to Table 4.5. It is important to remember that asthma severity is classified according to the worst parameter. Features to observe are respiratory rate, state of consciousness and whether the patient is able to speak in full sentences, in phrases or in words. All patients presenting to a doctor with an acute exacerbation of asthma must be assessed objectively for airflow obstruction by PEF measurement, or blood gas measurement if PEF measurement is not possible.

Management by the patient. Patients with asthma should have a personal written asthma action plan that provides information to aid recognition of an acute attack and lists treatment options (see Chapter 5). Action plans should include a crisis plan, and explain

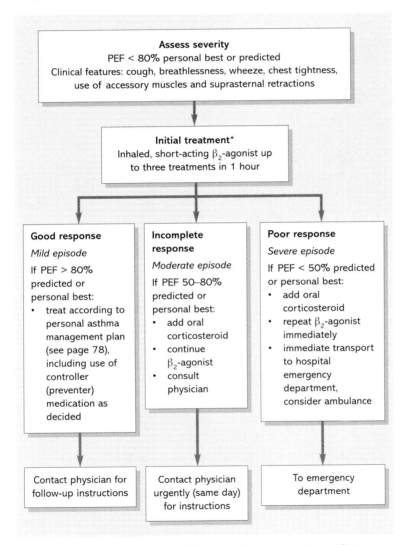

Figure 4.7 Algorithm for patients to follow in asthma exacerbations. *Patients at high risk of asthma-related death should contact a physician promptly after initial treatment as additional therapy may be required. PEF, peak expiratory flow.

when it is appropriate for a patient to call an ambulance. Plans must be written individually for each patient, but generally, patients should seek urgent medical help if they have used reliever medication three or more times without response, if they feel out of control, or if their PEF remains below 50% of predicted (Figure 4.7).

For less severe attacks that do not require hospital presentation, the first step is to increase regular bronchodilator therapy (however, frequent symptoms and frequent requirement for bronchodilator suggest that further treatment is needed). Less severe asthma attacks are diagnosed by frequent requirement for bronchodilator (up to once every 4 hours), night waking with asthma, and breathlessness. As a rule the PEF will be 50–80% predicted, the range depending on the person's previous asthma history. Oral corticosteroids, that is prednisolone, 1 mg/kg or 50 mg daily for adults, may be initiated by the patient in consultation with a local doctor. For those with more severe asthma, prompt access to a supply of oral corticosteroids is important to prevent severe exacerbations, and such patients may keep a store of these medications at home. Once commenced, oral corticosteroid therapy should continue for at least 5 days.

Hospital referral is indicated for all patients who have persisting severe asthma or symptoms despite oral corticosteroid therapy, or in those in whom asthma is severe (Figure 4.7). Patients with a past history of severe or brittle (unpredictable and severe) asthma, intensive care admission, difficulties in accessing care or psychosocial problems may require hospital referral at an earlier stage. Admission to hospital enables the administration of parenteral asthma therapy and observation of a patient with severe airflow obstruction to ensure that response to asthma treatment is occurring, thereby ensuring administration of therapy and patient safety. The hospital also provides an environment for ventilatory support if this is required.

Most deaths of people with asthma occur out of hospital, usually in those with severe chronic asthma, but also in some considered to have mild asthma. Treatment with bronchodilator medication in the absence of controller (preventer) treatments or overuse of bronchodilator medication is a particular risk factor for fatal asthma. Further risk factors are a previous life-threatening asthma attack, admission to hospital for asthma in the previous year and social or physical isolation from medical care, including psychosocial disability, especially psychiatric illness, substance abuse, poor treatment adherence and difficulty accessing treatment. Individuals with these features should be observed carefully and may require early referral to hospital.

Protective factors for asthma death are regular use of inhaled corticosteroids and possession of a personal written asthma management plan.

All patients who have been admitted to hospital with asthma should see a respiratory specialist. Those with life-threatening or brittle asthma should remain under the care of a specialist.

Treatment of acute severe asthma in hospital. Treatment of an acute exacerbation is based on the initial assessment of severity. Classification of severity depends on objective signs of airflow obstruction, including ability to talk in sentences, pulse rate, conscious state and, most importantly, PEF readings. Oxygen saturation measurements are useful, but it is important to remember that oxygen saturation may be elevated by oxygen administration with nebulized medication and does not reflect the adequacy of ventilation as determined by blood CO_2 measurements.

In the emergency department. The principles of acute asthma management in the emergency department are outlined in Figure 4.8. All patients should receive inhaled bronchodilator, and those with moderate or severe exacerbations should receive oral or parenteral corticosteroid therapy. For patients with life-threatening attacks, intensive care services should be sought. Patients not responding to treatment and stable within 2 hours should be considered for admission to hospital.

In hospital. Acute asthma management in hospital is summarized in Figure 4.9. Once a patient is admitted to hospital, monitoring

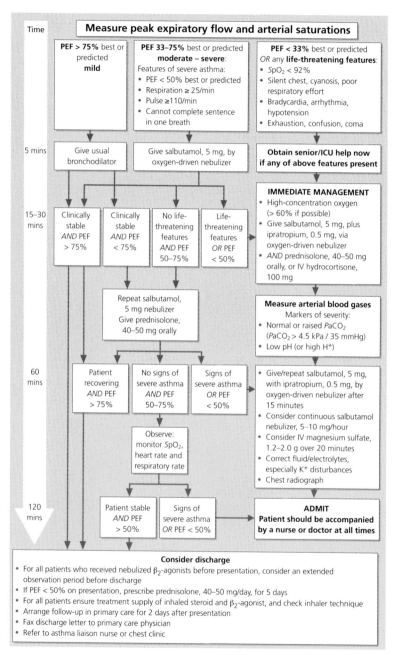

Figure 4.8 Acute asthma management in the emergency department. Adapted from British Thoracic Society/Scottish Intercollegiate Guidelines Network guideline.

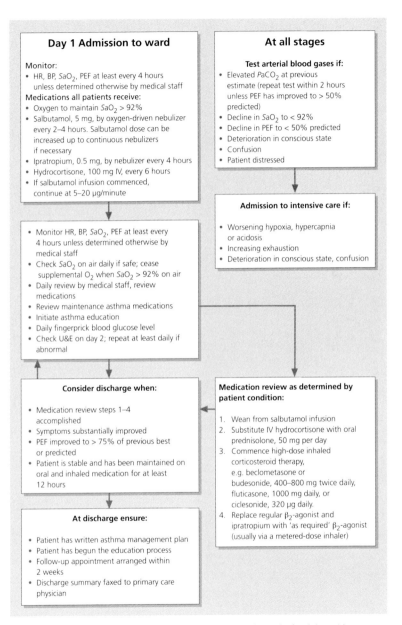

Day 1 Admission to ward

Monitor:
- HR, BP, SaO_2, PEF at least every 4 hours unless determined otherwise by medical staff

Medications all patients receive:
- Oxygen to maintain $SaO_2 > 92\%$
- Salbutamol, 5 mg, by oxygen-driven nebulizer every 2–4 hours. Salbutamol dose can be increased up to continuous nebulizers if necessary
- Ipratropium, 0.5 mg, by nebulizer every 4 hours
- Hydrocortisone, 100 mg IV, every 6 hours
- If salbutamol infusion commenced, continue at 5–20 µg/minute

---

- Monitor HR, BP, SaO_2, PEF at least every 4 hours unless determined otherwise by medical staff
- Check SaO_2 on air daily if safe; cease supplemental O_2 when $SaO_2 > 92\%$ on air
- Daily review by medical staff, review medications
- Review maintenance asthma medications
- Initiate asthma education
- Daily fingerprick blood glucose level
- Check U&E on day 2; repeat at least daily if abnormal

Consider discharge when:

- Medication review steps 1–4 accomplished
- Symptoms substantially improved
- PEF improved to > 75% of previous best or predicted
- Patient is stable and has been maintained on oral and inhaled medication for at least 12 hours

---

At discharge ensure:

- Patient has written asthma management plan
- Patient has begun the education process
- Follow-up appointment arranged within 2 weeks
- Discharge summary faxed to primary care physician

At all stages

Test arterial blood gases if:
- Elevated $PaCO_2$ at previous estimate (repeat test within 2 hours unless PEF has improved to > 50% predicted)
- Decline in SaO_2 to < 92%
- Decline in PEF to < 50% predicted
- Deterioration in conscious state
- Confusion
- Patient distressed

Admission to intensive care if:

- Worsening hypoxia, hypercapnia or acidosis
- Increasing exhaustion
- Deterioration in conscious state, confusion

Medication review as determined by patient condition:

1. Wean from salbutamol infusion
2. Substitute IV hydrocortisone with oral prednisolone, 50 mg per day
3. Commence high-dose inhaled corticosteroid therapy, e.g. beclometasone or budesonide, 400–800 mg twice daily, fluticasone, 1000 mg daily, or ciclesonide, 320 µg daily.
4. Replace regular β_2-agonist and ipratropium with 'as required' β_2-agonist (usually via a metered-dose inhaler)

Figure 4.9 Algorithm for management in the hospital ward of adults with acute asthma. BP, blood pressure; HR, heart rate; $PaCO_2$, partial pressure of oxygen in arterial blood; PEF, peak expiratory flow; SaO_2, oxygen saturation in arterial blood; SpO_2, SaO_2 estimated by pulse oximetry; U&E, urea and electrolytes.

and treatment should continue with:
- frequent (at least every 2 hours) observation of PEF, oxygen saturation, blood pressure and pulse
- oxygen administration to maintain oxygen saturation above 92%
- administration of β_2-agonists at least every 4 hours, and continuously if required
- administration of corticosteroid therapy orally or intravenously
- observation for deterioration in clinical state.

Ongoing review in hospital ensures recovery and introduces patients to their ongoing preventative medication and the management plan likely to be required following a hospital admission for asthma. The time in hospital presents an ideal opportunity for formal asthma education; interventions that provide in-hospital asthma education have shown benefits in terms of reduced re-admission rates.

Follow-up. All patients should leave hospital with medication, a written plan of what to do if their asthma worsens and a follow-up medical appointment for ongoing management. Oral corticosteroid therapy should be continued for at least 5 days following discharge. It is important that asthma control is assessed following a hospital admission and ongoing maintenance medication is adjusted accordingly.

What to do when recommended treatment fails

It is important that, in the event that asthma is poorly controlled using medication recommended in guidelines, treatment is not escalated without careful consideration of whether it is warranted. Three questions should be asked:
- Is the patient receiving the medication?
- Does the patient really have asthma?
- Does the patient have severe asthma?

Is the patient receiving the medication? Many obstacles exist to patients receiving their medication. It may be difficult to obtain for reasons of cost or inconvenience. It then has to be taken. Patients perform a 'cost–benefit' analysis as to whether to take the medication, an analysis that includes their beliefs about the benefits of the treatment and the likely outcome of their asthma, and their fears about drug side effects. The health professional must take part in this analysis and address issues that arise in order to aid adherence to a medication plan.

Patients then need to use their device effectively. Many people, especially the young and very old, find this difficult. A major part of consultation with a patient who is not successful in achieving good asthma control should be a review of inhaler use and technique, as this can be a significant barrier to medication effectiveness.

Does the patient really have asthma? Other diagnoses to consider have been listed in Figure 3.2. Any patient who does not respond to medication should undergo lung function testing to confirm the diagnosis. Physical examination may suggest that other investigations, such as a chest radiography, might be relevant. For children too young to perform spirometry reliably (usually less than 7 years), a specialist opinion should be sought if the diagnosis is uncertain, as the consequences in children of unnecessary inhaled corticosteroids (> 400 µg per day) can be significant.

Does the patient have severe asthma? A very few patients do have severe asthma that continues to be unstable despite demonstrated excellent medication use. Such people should be referred to specialist care as other pharmaceutical options are available. Long-term use of oral corticosteroids should be moderated by the use of steroid-sparing agents.

Key points – management

- Drugs used in the management of asthma can be classified as controllers (preventers) or relievers: controllers are taken daily on a long-term basis to control persistent asthma; relievers are used to reverse rapidly the bronchoconstriction and associated symptoms during acute attacks.
- Controllers (e.g. inhaled corticosteroids) are the mainstay of asthma therapy. Increasing use of relievers (short-acting β_2-agonists) indicates inadequate disease control.
- Asthma therapy should be tailored to disease severity; current management guidelines recommend a stepwise approach to treatment.
- All patients with asthma should have a written asthma action plan.
- Acute exacerbations of asthma usually respond well to inhaled β_2-agonists and a course of oral corticosteroid.
- If guideline treatment fails, adherence and diagnosis should be re-examined before treatment is escalated.

Key references

Barnes PJ, Pedersen S. The efficacy and safety of inhaled corticosteroids in asthma. *Am J Respir Dis* 1993; 148:S1–26.

British Thoracic Society, Scottish Intercollegiate Guidelines Network. British guideline on the management of asthma. *Thorax* 2003;58(suppl 1): i1–94.
www.sign.ac.uk/guidelines/fulltext/63/index.html
www.brit-thoracic.org.uk/asthma-guideline-download.html

Clark TJH, Godfrey S, Lee TH, eds. *Asthma*. London: Chapman and Hall Medical, 2000.

Gibson PG, Powell H, Coughlan J et al. Self-management education and regular practitioner review for adults with asthma. *Cochrane Database Syst Rev* 2002;issue 3. CD001117.
www.thecochranelibrary.com

National Heart, Lung, and Blood Institute at the National Institutes of Health, and the World Health Organization. *GINA Workshop Report, Global Strategy for Asthma Management and Prevention.* Bethesda: NIH/NHLBI, 2002 (publication number 02-3659).

Silverman M, ed. *Childhood Asthma and Other Wheezing Disorders.* London: Chapman and Hall, 1995.

www.ginasthma.com

Preventing asthma attacks from occurring is the most effective means of controlling asthma. This involves identifying and avoiding risk factors and triggers; in turn, this requires effective patient education and follow-up.

Patient partnerships

Included in the goals of good asthma management is the need to meet patients' goals and expectations as well as those of the health practitioners. Good asthma management means that a partnership should be established between the patient and health professional, with shared treatment goals noted in a jointly written and agreed self-management plan. This eases the pressure on health personnel resources and improves asthma outcomes.

Risk factor avoidance

Identification of risk factors that trigger asthma attacks and removal of the appropriate allergens and irritants from the patient's environment can reduce the frequency of symptoms and hospitalizations for asthma, and the need for medication. Appropriate avoidance behaviors are shown in Table 5.1. However, allergens should only be avoided when evidence (e.g. a positive skin-prick test) exists that the patient is indeed allergic to that specific allergen; if not, then allergen avoidance is not recommended.

House-dust mites are the most common source of domestic allergens. They breed fastest in damp, humid climates. Avoidance measures should be particularly directed at the patient's bedroom, but ideally the entire home should be treated. Bedlinen and blankets should be washed weekly in hot water, and mattresses and pillows protected by air-tight covers. Carpets and furnishing fabrics should be avoided wherever possible, and the bedroom should be well ventilated. Acaricides are of little use.

TABLE 5.1

Allergen and irritant avoidance

Allergen avoidance

House-dust mite

- Wash bedlinen and blankets once a week in hot water (> 55°C)
- Protect mattresses and pillows with air-tight covers
- Remove carpets, particularly in bedrooms
- Avoid fabric-covered furniture
- Wash curtains and soft toys
- If possible, use a vacuum cleaner with filters

Animal allergens

- Remove animals from house
- If removal of family pets is not possible or desirable, keep animals out of bedrooms and wash them regularly

Cockroach allergen

- Clean infected houses regularly
- Use pesticides (but ensure asthmatic patient is not present if pesticide sprays are used, and air house thoroughly before patient returns)

Fungal spores and pollens

- Close doors and windows and remain indoors when mould and pollen counts are highest
- Air conditioning can be helpful, provided unit is kept clean

General measures

Tobacco smoke

- Stop smoking
- Avoid smoking in rooms used by children with asthma
- Avoid public areas where people smoke

(CONTINUED)

TABLE 5.1 (CONTINUED)

Allergen and irritant avoidance

General measures

Indoor air pollutants

- Vent all furnaces and stoves to exterior
- Keep rooms well ventilated
- Avoid household sprays and polishes

Colds and other viral respiratory infections

- Patients with asthma should have annual influenza vaccination
- When cold symptoms appear, treat with inhaled short-acting β_2-agonist, introduce oral corticosteroids early, or increase inhaled corticosteroid dose if asthma status deteriorates
- Continue anti-inflammatory treatment for several weeks to ensure adequate control

Physical activity

- Should not be avoided, but appropriate medication is necessary:
  - pretreat with short- or long-acting β_2-agonist or cromoglicate before exercising
  - training and warm-up exercises can reduce symptoms

Animal allergens. A pet in the home to which the patient with asthma is allergic is a major risk factor for current asthma symptoms. Ideally, such pets – usually cats – should be removed from the home, but this may not be acceptable. If animals cannot be removed, they should be kept away from bedrooms; weekly washing of the pet appears to reduce the allergen load.

Cockroach allergen is a major cause of asthma in some areas. It can be reduced by regular cleaning of the home and by the use of pesticides. If pesticide sprays are used, however, the patient should not be present while spraying is in progress, and the home should be aired thoroughly before the patient returns.

Molds and pollens. The number of fungal spores can be reduced by removing or cleaning mold-infested objects. A low humidity (less than 50%) is important, and so a dehumidifier or air conditioning may be useful; such devices should be cleaned regularly. Exposure to outdoor allergens, such as pollens, can be minimized by keeping doors and windows closed, and by remaining indoors as much as possible during high-risk periods.

Smoking. Passive smoking increases the risk of allergic sensitization in children, and worsens the frequency and severity of symptoms in asthmatic children. Parents of such children should be advised not to smoke and to prohibit smoking in rooms used by their children.

Indoor pollutants. Common indoor pollutants include nitrogen dioxide, carbon monoxide and particles. Adequate ventilation and maintenance of heating systems are the most effective measures for reducing exposure to such pollutants.

Occupational exposure. Early identification of occupational sensitizers and removal of the patient from further exposure are important elements in the management of occupational asthma.

Food allergy is a rare cause of asthma exacerbations, and occurs mainly in young children. Individuals with severe food allergies should avoid the food in question and be assessed by an allergy specialist. Clear evidence of IgE immunoreactivity to the food or a positive double-blind food challenge should be obtained to justify and clarify the role of ongoing food avoidance. Patients with asthma and severe food allergies causing anaphylaxis are at particular risk of death. They should be well educated in avoidance of the specific food and should have access to injectable epinephrine (adrenaline).

Aspirin intolerance is an important cause of worsening asthma in adults. Patients who are affected should be advised to avoid all NSAIDs except those selective against cyclooxygenase 2 (Cox-2 inhibitors).

Immunotherapy

Specific immunotherapy, aimed at treating the underlying allergy, has been shown to be effective in patients with asthma caused by house-dust mite, grass or other pollens, animal dander or *Alternaria*. Such treatment may be useful in patients for whom allergen avoidance is not possible or whose symptoms are not controlled by conventional medication. Since immunotherapy is relatively contraindicated in those with unstable asthma and those with abnormal lung function, it is practically limited to those with milder disease, especially those who suffer from allergic rhinitis. There is some evidence that immunotherapy can prevent the progression of allergic rhinitis to asthma.

Immunotherapy should only be undertaken by healthcare professionals with specific training in the diagnosis of allergy and the management of anaphylaxis.

Asthma management plans

Education is essential to enable patients to make the decisions needed to control their asthma. This involves the preparation of a detailed management plan (Table 5.2), which is agreed between the

TABLE 5.2

Elements of an asthma management plan

- The daily dose of long-term preventive medication needed to control asthma and prevent symptoms
- Specific triggers to avoid
- What to do if asthma worsens:
  - name and dose of bronchodilator to be taken immediately for quick relief of symptoms
  - how to recognize deteriorating control (e.g. increasing cough, chest tightness or breathing difficulties, nocturnal symptoms, increasing use of quick-acting reliever medicine)
  - how to treat worsening asthma, and what to do if a cold develops
  - how and when to seek medical attention

patient and the physician, and is tailored to the needs and circumstances of the individual patient. Symptom-based and PEF-based plans have been shown to be equally effective. Plans should be written down so patients can refer to them (Figures 5.1 and 5.2).

A zone system, which classifies the level of asthma control according to symptoms and PEF (if available), is a useful feature of management plans. This approach helps patients to understand the chronic and variable nature of asthma, monitor their condition, identify signs of deteriorating control, and take appropriate action.

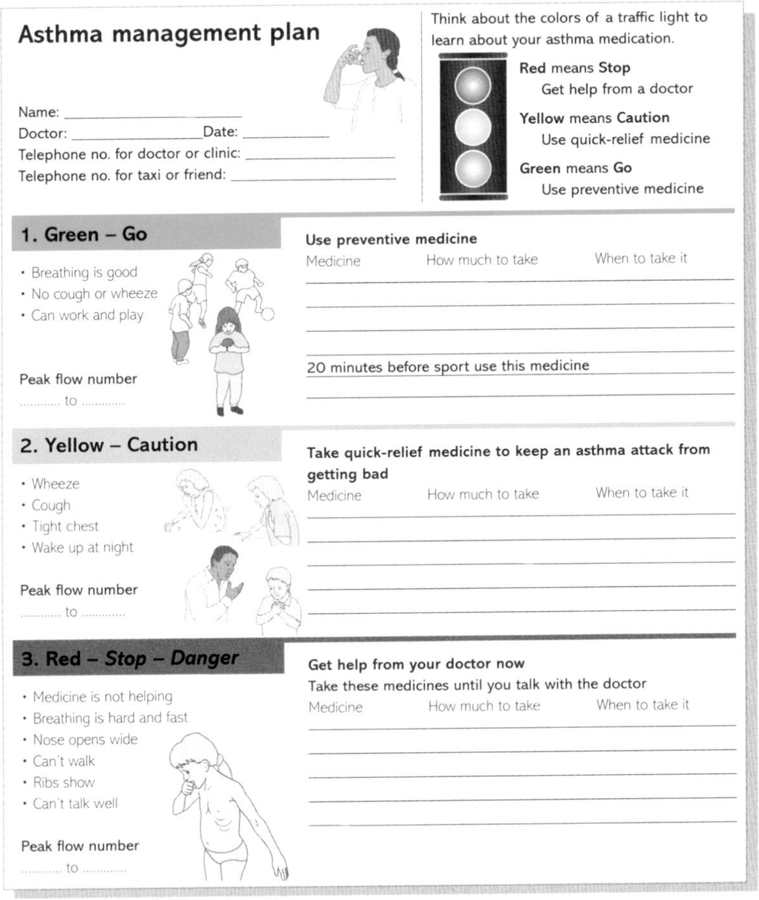

Asthma management plan

Name: _____
Doctor: _____ Date: _____
Telephone no. for doctor or clinic: _____
Telephone no. for taxi or friend: _____

Think about the colors of a traffic light to learn about your asthma medication.

Red means **Stop**
   Get help from a doctor
Yellow means **Caution**
   Use quick-relief medicine
Green means **Go**
   Use preventive medicine

1. Green – Go

- Breathing is good
- No cough or wheeze
- Can work and play

Peak flow number
.... to ....

Use preventive medicine
Medicine   How much to take   When to take it

20 minutes before sport use this medicine

2. Yellow – Caution

- Wheeze
- Cough
- Tight chest
- Wake up at night

Peak flow number
.... to ....

Take quick-relief medicine to keep an asthma attack from getting bad
Medicine   How much to take   When to take it

3. Red – Stop – Danger

- Medicine is not helping
- Breathing is hard and fast
- Nose opens wide
- Can't walk
- Ribs show
- Can't talk well

Peak flow number
.... to ....

Get help from your doctor now
Take these medicines until you talk with the doctor
Medicine   How much to take   When to take it

Figure 5.1 Asthma management plans can be based on a zone system, which details the action needed to control asthma at different levels of severity.

In the management plan shown in Figure 5.1, the three zones correspond to the colors of a traffic light.

- The green zone indicates 'all clear'. Asthma is controlled, with few symptoms (less than two a week) and no interference with everyday life; PEF is 80–100% of personal best and PEF variability is less than 20%. Moving to a lower treatment step can be considered if the patient remains in this zone for at least 3 months.
- The yellow zone indicates that caution is necessary. Mild symptoms are present and PEF is 60–80% of personal best with 20–30% variability. This may indicate an acute attack requiring a temporary increase in medication, or an overall deterioration that requires additional treatment.
- The red zone indicates an emergency. Asthma symptoms are present at rest and may interfere with activity; PEF is below 60% of personal best. Immediate intervention is necessary.

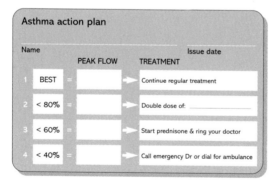

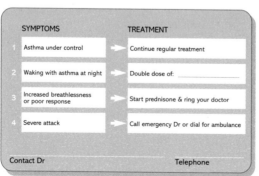

Figure 5.2
A credit-card-sized asthma self-management plan. This plan has been evaluated in clinical trials and introduced in several countries.

Another management plan, the credit-card-sized document shown in Figure 5.2, has been evaluated in clinical trials, and has been successfully introduced in several countries, including the UK, New Zealand and Australia.

Promoting adherence. If patients do not adhere to their medication and management plan, their asthma will not be controlled effectively, yet in adherence studies, less than 50% of patients take their medication as prescribed. Causes of non-adherence may or may not be related to medication (Table 5.3).

Regular consultations are necessary to give patients an opportunity to talk about their concerns, needs and expectations in relation to their asthma and its treatment. Action can then be taken to address any problems identified, and to resolve any fears or concerns that patients may have. Strategies for encouraging adherence are listed in Table 5.4. Together the patient and the healthcare professional can identify joint goals of treatment, such as 'staying out of hospital' or 'playing football', that are relevant to the patient and therefore likely to promote adherence. Thus, at each visit, the physician should check:

- whether the stated goals have been achieved
- adherence to, and concerns about, medication and the management plan
- the patient's use of the controller (preventer) and reliever inhalers, PEF meter or other devices
- need for emergency attendances
- avoidance of triggers.

Once control has been achieved, regular follow-up at 1–6-month intervals as appropriate is necessary to assess whether the management plan is meeting its objectives. This includes review of:

- nocturnal symptoms
- effect of symptoms on normal activity
- use of reliever rescue medication
- need for urgent medical attention
- normal PEF.

TABLE 5.3

Factors leading to non-adherence with asthma therapy

Medication-related factors

- Misunderstanding the need for both long-term and short-acting drugs
- Complicated treatment regimens
- Difficulty in giving medicine to young children
- Difficulty using inhalers
- Adverse effects
- Fear of adverse effects or addiction
- Cost
- Dislike of medication
- Distance to pharmacies

Non-medication factors

- Disbelief or denial of cause of symptoms or attacks
- Misunderstanding of management plan
- Lack of guidance for self-management
- Dissatisfaction with healthcare professionals
- Unexpressed or undiscussed fears or concerns
- Inappropriate expectations
- Poor supervision, training or follow-up
- Cultural issues (traditions, beliefs about asthma and its treatment)
- Family issues (e.g. smoking, pets)

When to refer. In general, most patients with mild or moderate
asthma can be adequately managed in the primary care setting.

Referral to a specialist is advisable for patients with moderate or
severe persistent asthma, or if there are complicating conditions or
circumstances (Table 5.5). Children needing more than 400 µg
inhaled corticosteroids per day and adults needing more than
1000 µg per day with poor symptom control should also be
referred to a specialist.

TABLE 5.4

Strategies for improving adherence to asthma treatment

- Enquire about adherence to medication (patients are generally honest in admitting non-adherence)
- Educate patients and their families about the inflammatory basis of asthma and the need for ongoing treatments
- Enquire about and address concerns regarding medications and their use
- Identify and, if possible, address barriers to medication use (e.g. cost, knowledge of how to use the devices)
- Ask about family and cultural beliefs
- Encourage the patient in self-management
- Keep medication regimens simple – twice a day maximum
- Plan for reminders to use medication such as alarms, mobile phones
- Explain likely side effects and how to prevent them
- Be positive about the outcomes of treatments

TABLE 5.5

Situations requiring specialist referral for asthma

- Life-threatening attacks
- Moderate or severe persistent asthma
- Patient is unable to cope with self-management
- Atypical signs or symptoms, or difficulties with differential diagnosis
- Complicating conditions such as sinusitis, nasal polyposis, aspergillosis or severe rhinitis
- Further diagnostic tests required (e.g. provocation testing or complete lung function tests)
- Patient does not respond optimally to treatment
- Additional guidance needed (e.g. trigger avoidance or treatment complications)

Key points – prevention of asthma attacks

- Preventing asthma attacks from occurring is the most effective means of controlling asthma.
- Identification of risk factors that trigger asthma attacks and removal of the appropriate allergens and irritants from the patient's environment can reduce the frequency of symptoms and hospitalizations for asthma, and decrease the need for medication.
- Immunotherapy is helpful in some patients in whom specific allergens can be shown to be causative, in whom allergen avoidance is not possible or whose symptoms are not controlled by conventional medication.
- A written self-management plan empowers patients to manage their asthma optimally.
- Failure to respond to treatment may result from non-adherence to the prescribed treatment. Attention must be paid to the patients' ability to take their inhaled therapy correctly.
- Adherence to medications is a major challenge to both healthcare practitioners and patients. Identifying problems surounding care and creating a patient partnership with agreed treatment goals can facilitate adherence.

Key references

Abramson MJ, Puy RM, Weiner JM. Allergen immunotherapy for asthma. *Cochrane Database Syst Rev* 2003;issue 4. CD001186. www.thecochranelibrary.com

Bousquet J, Lockey R, Malling HJ. Allergen immunotherapy: therapeutic vaccines for allergic diseases. A WHO position paper. *J Allergy Clin Immunol* 1998;102:558–62.

Fishwick D, Beasley R. Use of peak flow-based self-management plans by adult asthmatic patients. *Eur Respir J* 1996;9:861–5.

National Heart, Lung, and Blood Institute at the National Institutes of Health, and the World Health Organization. *GINA Workshop Report, Global Strategy for Asthma Management and Prevention.* Bethesda:NIH/NHLBI, 2002 (publication number 02-3659).

www.ginasthma.com

As many as 80% of people with asthma will develop exercise-induced symptoms, so that exercise for some people is a noticeable trigger for asthma. Indeed, in some people asthma is only evident on exercising, particularly in children, in whom the benefits of exercise are particularly important. Consequently, managing exercise-induced asthma and enabling individuals to exercise despite asthma is an important part of asthma management.

In addition, the issue of asthma in elite sporting activities has risen to prominence. In some Olympic teams as many as 20% of athletes declare that they have asthma, raising concerns about the appropriate use of anti-asthma medications in this group. Optimizing asthma diagnosis and treatment in elite athletes is critical to optimizing performance and deserves particular attention.

Diagnosis

Exercise-induced asthma is defined as a transient increase in airway resistance that follows vigorous exercise. Many people complain of shortness of breath while exercising, and this symptom is often magnified in people with asthma. Typically, people with asthma describe developing wheeze, shortness of breath and sometimes cough both during and, more importantly, after exercise. For some individuals with brittle asthma, the response to exercise can be severe, and may be a strong disincentive to exercise.

Exercise-induced asthma appears to be more common in those with atopy and to be seen more often on exercise in very cold weather.

A feature of exercise-induced asthma is a refractory period, whereby induction of exercise-induced asthma appears to be protective for further episodes for a period of several hours. Thus, individuals who experience a bout of exercise-induced asthma can undertake subsequent exercise with relative protection from further episodes. This refractory period can be inhibited by anti-inflammatory medications such as indomethacin.

In the laboratory or for research, exercise-induced asthma can be brought on by a short period (6–8 minutes) of high-intensity exercise of at least 70% of maximum predicted capacity. Lung function is measured following this exercise; a decline in FEV_1 of more than 10% from baseline denotes a diagnosis of exercise-induced asthma (Figure 6.1).

The problem with laboratory exercise tests is that they may not replicate the environmental conditions under which exercise is performed; for example neither the temperature nor the humidity of ambient air is likely to be the same as that encountered during outdoor exercise. In addition, it is often difficult to achieve adequately high workloads for very fit individuals such as athletes using laboratory exercise equipment. Hence field testing can be undertaken to make the diagnosis, which requires recording of PEF or lung function following exercise in the field. However, this too is subject to varying conditions of humidity, temperature and conduct

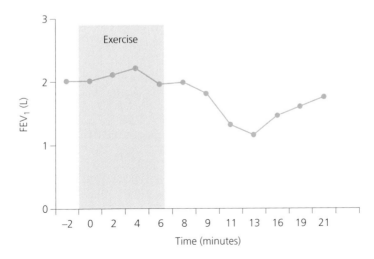

Figure 6.1 Exercise challenge testing: during brief, high-intensity exercise, lung function transiently improves, but in people with exercise-induced asthma, lung function is likely to fall in the minutes following exercise.

of the test, rendering standardization difficult. As a consequence of these difficulties, surrogate challenges for exercise-induced asthma have been developed.

Airway challenge testing can be categorized into direct and indirect airway responses (Figure 6.2). Indirect challenges cause bronchoconstriction by stimulating airway mast cells to release mediator and thereby cause secondary airway smooth-muscle constriction. Direct challenges act pharmacologically on the airway smooth muscle to cause airway narrowing.

Indirect challenges. Exercise challenge testing is an indirect challenge relying on airway responses to exercise, such as airway drying and cooling, to cause smooth-muscle contraction. Because of the difficulties of replicating field exercise in the laboratory to achieve consistency of diagnosis, a number of surrogate challenges for exercise have been developed. Chief among these is the eucapnic voluntary hyperventilation challenge, in which the subject is asked to breathe a mixture of dry air with 5% CO_2 at 85% of their maximal ventilation (approximately 30 times FEV_1) for 6 minutes, and their FEV_1 is monitored after challenge. This surrogate challenge has been shown to correlate very well with actual exercise

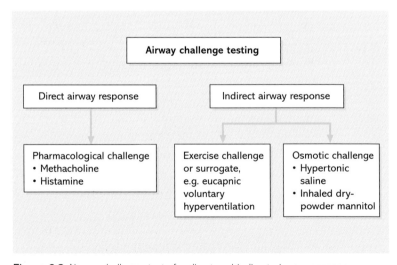

Figure 6.2 Airway challenge tests for direct and indirect airway responses.

challenge and is suitable for use by athletes. A fall in FEV_1 of 10% following the eucapnic voluntary hyperventilation challenge has been adopted by the International Olympic Committee as the preferred criterion for confirmation of an asthma diagnosis in elite athletes.

Indirect airway challenges such as mannitol and hypertonic saline have been shown to correlate very well with eucapnic voluntary hyperventilation challenges. These agents mimic the dehydration of the airways that is probably responsible for exercise-induced asthma (see Mechanisms, below).

Direct challenges. Most individuals with airway hyperresponsiveness to methacholine will yield a positive result to exercise challenge. However, some, particularly elite athletes, will have a positive surrogate exercise challenge result despite negative direct airway challenge test results. It is therefore important not to exclude exercise-induced asthma on the basis of a negative direct airway challenge test result.

Mechanisms

During inhalation air is humidified and warmed to body temperature. At rest, this process usually occurs in the upper airways, particularly in the nose. During exercise, ventilation is increased, sometimes to levels exceeding 100 L/min, so that the individual has to breathe through the mouth to overcome upper airway resistance. Mouth breathing and increased ventilation lead to the lower airways being recruited to warm and humidify inspired air, resulting in progressive evaporation of airway surface fluid and hyperosmolarity of this fluid. It is thought that hyperosmolarity of the airway surface fluid provokes mast-cell degranulation, which can then stimulate airway narrowing through smooth-muscle contraction. In support of these theories, exercise-induced asthma has been shown to correlate with increased blood mast-cell mediators. In addition, breathing humidified, warmed air during exercise has been shown to be protective for the development of exercise-induced bronchoconstriction. Swimming is often recommended as exercise to people with asthma, as inspiration will occur from the humidified air near the water surface, decreasing the dehydrating stimulus to the lower airways.

By contrast, many individuals with asthma find cold air a potent trigger of symptoms. This is because the water content of air is temperature-dependent, cold air holding less water than warmer air. Thus, exercise in the cold, such as skiing, requires greater water transfer for complete saturation of inspired air than does exercise in warmer climates, and cold, dry air is therefore a more potent stimulus for developing exercise-induced asthma.

Exercise-induced symptoms appear to be more common in atopic individuals; this observation may imply that inhaled allergens play a role. In particular, loss of the protective functions of the upper airways during inspiration may permit increased penetration to the lower respiratory tract of allergens and other particles likely to stimulate asthma. Although this has not been proved to be a cause in laboratory-induced exercise-induced asthma, increased lower airway exposure to allergens and extremes of environmental changes such as heat and cold may be particularly relevant in elite athletes who spend a large amount of time training with high ventilation, thereby increasing their cumulative exposure to such potential triggers.

Exercise-induced asthma in athletes

The high prevalence of exercise-induced asthma in elite athletes is a recently recognized problem. Escalating use of bronchodilator treatments by elite athletes has prompted rulings from the International Olympic Committee. Some elite cold-weather athletes, such as cross-country skiers, will develop exercise-induced asthma, so called 'skier's asthma'. In summer athletes, a high occurrence of asthma has been reported in elite swimmers. In both these instances, training for prolonged periods at high ventilatory workloads and consequent large exposure to very cold or chlorinated air, respectively, is thought to contribute to an airway injury that may lead to exercise-induced asthma. The finding that older athletes and those from sports that are predominantly aerobic are more likely to have exercise-induced asthma supports this theory.

The symptoms of elite athletes with asthma are thought to differ from those of non-athletes in that they may complain of poor performance or fatigue rather than dyspnea. Investigation of symptoms of elite athletes revealed that traditional asthma symptoms have a sensitivity of only 60% in predicting exercise-induced bronchoconstriction in laboratory challenge. Thus, poor performance in an athlete ought to prompt consideration of exercise-induced asthma.

Treatment

Treatment for exercise-induced asthma in those with pre-existing asthma is determined by evaluating lung function and symptoms. Individuals with lung function abnormalities and symptoms of asthma both with and without exercise should have the usual controller (preventer) medication prescribed. Inhaled corticosteroids have been shown to be very effective in reducing airway hyperresponsiveness both generally and following exercise. However, many people with asthma do have asthma symptoms despite regular use of inhaled corticosteroids and may require additional short-acting β_2-agonists before exercise to prevent exercise-induced asthma.

Some individuals with normal interval lung function complain of symptoms only on exercise. Although regular preventative treatment may be appropriate for such people if exercise is very frequent, it may be reasonable to use short-acting β_2-agonists to prevent exercise-induced bronchoconstriction in those who experience symptoms only episodically, such as less than twice a week. Additional or alternative treatments may be required in some, and include mast-cell stabilizers, such as cromoglicate or nedocromil, or leukotriene modifiers, such as montelukast.

Non-drug strategies for the treatment of exercise-induced asthma rely on the refractory period that follows induction of airway narrowing with exercise. It is frequently recommended that athletes with exercise-induced asthma warm up slowly. They may institute strategies such as repeated high-intensity runs during a warm-up to prevent exercise-induced asthma occurring in the main competition.

Key points – exercise-induced asthma

- Exercise-induced asthma is defined as a transient increase in airway resistance that follows vigorous exercise.
- It appears to be more common in those with atopy and to be seen more often on exercise in very cold weather.
- Induction of exercise-induced asthma appears to be protective for further episodes for a period of several hours.
- Exercise testing or other direct or indirect challenges are used in diagnosis.
- In elite athletes, direct airway challenges may not reveal exercise-induced asthma, so indirect surrogate challenges must be used to confirm diagnosis.
- First-line treatment of exercise-induced asthma is inhaled corticosteroids to reduce airway hyperresponsiveness, with additional short-acting β_2-agonists before exercise if necessary.

Key reference

Holzer K, Anderson SD, Douglass J. Exercise in elite summer athletes: Challenges for diagnosis. *J Allergy Clin Immunol* 2002;110:374–80.

Immunologic treatments

The incidences of allergy and asthma in developing countries have increased with the acquisition of westernized lifestyles. It has been suggested that these increases correspond with the decreasing incidence of childhood infections; as children are not exposed to the immunostimulatory effects of these infections, the stimulation necessary for the production of immunomodulatory T cells and interferon-γ is lacking. This 'hygiene hypothesis' is supported by the recent finding that respiratory infections in early infancy, such as measles, protect against the development of allergy. Further evidence to support this hypothesis comes from the inverse relationship that is being found between the magnitude of the response to BCG (bacille Calmette–Guérin) in the first year of life and the development of allergy in asthma later in childhood. Thus, by administering a strong stimulus to interferon-γ early in life, such as *Mycobacterium vaccae*, it may be possible to rectify any defect in interferon-γ production and, therefore, prevent the onset and progression of allergic tissue responses.

A new immunologic approach to controlling asthma has recently been described using a humanized monoclonal antibody against IgE, which is administered on a 2–4-weekly basis by subcutaneous injection. This monoclonal antibody (omalizumab) binds to the part of the IgE molecule that attaches to the high-affinity and low-affinity receptors on mediator-secreting cells, thereby depriving the cells of the necessary allergen-specific IgE required to trigger secretion of mediators. The net result of this treatment is that the serum level of IgE drops steeply with the first injection, and then gradually, over several weeks, IgE in the airways also falls in parallel with the loss of IgE receptors. Thus, after several months of treatment with omalizumab, both early- and late-phase allergen-induced bronchoconstriction is ablated in parallel with a reduction in airway inflammation, including a dramatic rise in tissue eosinophils. Clinical trials conducted for up to 2 years have revealed that this anti-allergy treatment is effective in the management of severe and chronic asthma, especially in reducing exacerbations and corticosteroid use. Omalizumab is now available in Australia and the USA, and would seem to be a particularly promising therapeutic approach for those patients with intransigent allergic asthma that fails to respond to conventional treatment.

Other approaches that look promising in the management of chronic severe asthma include:

- biological agents that block the effects of tumor necrosis factor (TNF)-α (e.g. soluble TNF-α receptor or monoclonal antibodies that can block TNF-α)
- selective antagonists for chemokine receptors (CCR), especially CCR3, which is involved in the recruitment of mast cells and eosinophils into the inflamed airways
- selective type-4 phosphodiesterase inhibitors, which have an anti-inflammatory action on a variety of inflammatory cells implicated in asthma pathogenesis and in addition exert some effect in relaxing airway smooth muscle.

In addition, intensive research is focused on developing a safer form of inhaled corticosteroid that interferes with the inflammatory pathways underpinning the pathogenesis of asthma and yet does not produce attendant side effects.

Genetic targeting

As treatments become more geared towards total prevention and cure of asthma, it is likely that they will focus not on broad populations, but on individuals who are at specific genetic risk. Identifying asthma susceptibility in genes is almost a growth industry at present. Although certain genes have been identified that increase the risk either of having asthma or of having more severe disease, it is likely that many more will be found that are more important and are, therefore, of direct relevance in selecting patients for appropriate treatments.

The results of genetic studies are also likely to have an impact on the drug treatment of asthma, as polymorphisms involving cellular receptors or enzyme pathways against which drugs are directed may influence their effectiveness (pharmacogenetics).

Hence, the future looks most promising for patients with asthma but, until new treatments are developed, it is essential that we make better use of the drugs currently available.

Key references

Barnes PJ. Cytokine-directed therapies for the treatment of chronic airway diseases. *Cytokine Growth Factor Rev* 2003:14:511–22.

Blease K, Lewis A, Raymon HK. Emerging treatments for asthma. *Expert Opin Emerg Drugs* 2003; 8:71–81.

Bush RK. The use of anti-IGgE in the treatment of allergic asthma. *Med Clin N Am* 2002;86(5):1113–29.

Erin EM, Williams TJ, Barnes PJ, Hansel TT. Eotaxin receptor (CCR3) antagonism in asthma and allergic disease. *Curr Drug Targets Inflamm Allergy* 2002;1:201–14.

Grootendorst DC, Rabe KF. Selective phosphodiesterase inhibitors for the treatment of asthma and chronic obstructive pulmonary disease. *Curr Opin Allergy Clin Immunol* 2002;2:61–7.

Useful resources

Global Initiative for Asthma (GINA)
www.ginasthma.com

International Union Against
Tuberculosis and Lung Disease
68 Boulevard Saint Michel
75006 Paris, France
Tel: +33 (0)1 44 32 03 60
Fax: +33 (0)1 43 29 90
www.iuatld.org

European Federation of Allergy
and Airways Diseases Patients'
Associations
www.efanet.org

European Academy of Allergology
and Clinical Immunology
www.eaaci.net

American Lung Association
Tel: 1 800 586 4872
www.lungusa.org

American Academy of Allergy,
Asthma & Immunology
611 East Wells Street
Milwaukee, WI 53202, USA
Tel: +1 414 272 6071
Patient advice: 1 800 822 2762
Fax: +1 414 272 6070
info@aaaai.org
www.aaaai.org

Asthma and Allergy Foundation of
America (AAFA)
1233 20th Street, NW, Suite 402
Washington, DC 20036, USA
Tel: +1 202 466 7643 /
1 800 7 ASTHMA
Fax: +1 202 466 8940
info@aafa.org
www.aafa.org

American Association for
Respiratory Care
9425 N MacArthur Blvd, Suite 100
Irving, TX 75063-4706, USA
Tel: +1 972 243 2272
Fax: +1 972 484 2720/6010
info@aarc.org
www.aarc.org

Allergy & Asthma Network
Mothers of Asthmatics (USA)
2751 Prosperity Ave, Suite 150
Fairfax, VA 22031, USA
Tel: 1 800 878 4403
Fax: +1 703 573 7794
www.aanma.org

US Environmental Protection
Agency
www.epa.gov/asthma/

Asthma UK
Summit House
70 Wilson Street
London EC2A 2DB
Tel: +44 (0)20 7226 2260
Helpline: 0845 7 01 02 03
Fax: +44 (0)20 7704 0740
www.asthma.org.uk

National Asthma Campaign Scotland
2a North Charlotte Street
Edinburgh EH2 4HR
Tel: +44 (0)131 226 2544
Fax: +44 (0)131 226 2401

British Lung Foundation
73–75 Goswell Road
London EC1V 7ER
Tel: +44 (0)20 7688 5555
Fax: +44 (0)20 7688 5556
enquiries@blf-uk.org
www.britishlungfoundation.com

British Thoracic Society
17 Doughty Street
London WC1N 2PL
Tel: +44 (0)20 7831 8778
Fax: +44 (0)20 7831 8766
bts@brit-thoracic.org.uk
www.brit-thoracic.org.uk

Scottish Intercollegiate Guidelines Network (SIGN)
www.sign.ac.uk/guidelines/fulltext/63/index.html

Canadian Lung Association
3 Raymond Street, Suite 300
Ottawa, ON   K1R 1A3
Tel: +1 613 569 6411
or 1 888 566 LUNG (5864)
Fax: +1 613 569 8860
info@lung.ca
www.lung.ca

Thoracic Society of Australia & New Zealand
145 Macquarie Street
Sydney NSW 2000
Tel: +61 (0)2 9256 5457
Fax: +61 (0)2 9241 4162
admin@thoracic.org.au
www.thoracic.org.au

National Asthma Council Australia
1 Palmerston Crescent
South Melbourne VIC 3205
Tel: +61 (0)3 9214 1476
Hotline: 1 800 032 495
Fax: +61 (0)3 9214 1400
nac@nationalasthma.org.au
www.nationalasthma.org.au

Asthma and Respiratory Foundation of New Zealand
Level 9, Clayton Ford House
132 The Terrace
PO Box 1459, Wellington
Tel: +64 (0)4 499 4592
Fax: +64 (0)4 499 4594
arf@asthmanz.co.nz
www.asthmanz.co.nz

Index

What the reviewers say:

This is a welcome extension to the Fast Facts series...
It provides easily accessible information
in a user-friendly fashion

On *Fast Facts – Inflammatory Bowel Disease*, 2nd edn, in *Doody's Health Sciences Review*, Aug 2006
(Winner of the BMA Medical Book Award for Gastroenterology, 2006)

I highly recommend this book to any clinician interested in what
important changes the past year has brought to psychiatry

On *Fast Facts – Psychiatry Highlights 2005–06*,
in *Doody's Health Sciences Review*, Aug 2006

perhaps the best source of practical guidance
on infant nutrition for all healthcare staff

On *Fast Facts – Infant Nutrition*, in *Nutrition and Dietetics*, June 2006

This is a book you will want to have

On *Fast Facts – Renal Disorders*,
in *EDTNA/ERCA Journal*, XXXII(1), 2006

the only book available that provides such a concise and
pertinent presentation on bladder cancer and its management

On *Fast Facts – Bladder Cancer*, 2nd edn, in *Doody's Health Sciences Review*, June 2006

I, for one, will make it part of
the mandatory reading for all my
respiratory registrars

On *Fast Facts – Obstructive Sleep Apnea*,
in *Australasian Sleep Association Newsletter*, December 2005

the entire book can be read as a crash course in less than two hours,
yet it does not ignore the complexity of human sexuality

On *Fast Facts – Sexual Dysfunction*, in
Journal of Nervous and Mental Disease, 193(6), 2005

quite simply, a terrific little book...
a fount of evidence-based wisdom

On *Fast Facts – Smoking Cessation*, in *Medical Journal of Australia*, 182(12), 2005

succeeds in delivering expert reviews of current research in the field
in a concise, reader-friendly format... I look forward to reading the
previous six editions and eagerly anticipate
the arrival of the next one in 2006.

On *Fast Facts – Vascular Surgery Highlights 2004–05*, in *Doody's Health Sciences Review*, 2005

This book is a little goldmine and
is very good value for money

On *Fast Facts – Endometriosis, 2nd edn*, in *Medical Journal of Australia*, 2004

concise and well written and accompanied by numerous excellent color
illustrations... an excellent little book! Score: 100 - 5 Stars

On *Fast Facts – Sexual Dysfunction*
in *Doody's Health Sciences Review*, 2004

this small volume is pleasingly pithy, erudite and
accessible, as well as being helpfully informative

On *Fast Facts – Bipolar Disorder, 2nd edn*, in *Medical Journal of Australia*, 2004

a timely and accessible book...
a worthwhile and handy tool for medical students

On *Fast Facts – Dyspepsia*, in *Digestive and Liver Disease*, 36, 2004

provides a lot of information in a concise and easily accessible format...
a practical guide to managing most lower respiratory tract infections

On *Fast Facts – Respiratory Tract Infection*, in *Respiratory Care*, 49(1), 2004

www.fastfacts.com

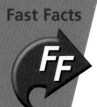

Fast Facts

Imagine if every time
you wanted to know something
you knew where to look ...

Fast Facts

... you do now

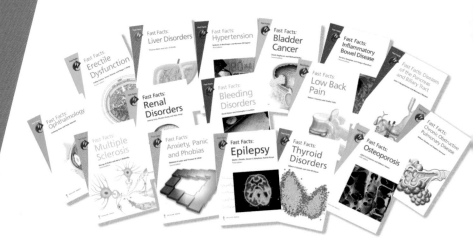

- *Fast Facts* – compact, evidence-based guides designed to help you improve patient care

- Practical, dependable information from experts of international standing

- Concise text, accessible design and comprehensive illustration so that key clinical facts stand out from the page

Orders

For a complete list of books, to order via the website or to find regional distributors, please go to
www.fastfacts.com

For telephone orders, please call +44 (0)1752 202301 (Europe),
1 800 247 6553 (USA, toll free) or +1 419 281 1802 (Americas)